WEIG DILEMMA ~~FOR WOMEN~~ OVER 40 YEARS:

THE OVER 40 WOMEN'S GUIDE TO SEXY BODIES

Tiehu Clarke

Tiehu M. Clarke

8220 Sunrise Lakes Blvd, Blvd 57,

Sunrise, FL, 33322

9547093384

Smartg7@hotmail.com

Weight loss dilemma over 40

by

Tiehu Clarke

Introduction

Thank you for choosing my book. By the time you hit your 40s, you've probably hit a few bumps in the road. Well, maybe more than a few. The result? You've got more confidence, don't care as much as what people think, and have a good grip on who it is you are.

And if that's not fabulous, I don't know what is.

So what if some things aren't quite the same in your body as they used to be? Would you want to go back to your life when you were in your 20s just because your tummy was flatter and you didn't have the so-called "old lady" arm waggle? No way!

You can still have a great looking body AND all the confidence that being over 40 brings. What could be better than that?

This book is all about getting your body and your sexy back. Being over 40 means that you've probably realized that not everything in life is perfect and that means your body too. But things that are imperfect can often be the most beautiful. And no one has the perfect body, no matter what their age. But that doesn't mean that you can't look and feel fabulous. You absolutely can. You've just got to commit yourself.

It's time to get your sexy back. Let's get started!!!

Whether you are just getting started by working out for the first time, getting back into it after some off-months (or years), or you have been active for your entire life, and you're just looking for something new and different, welcome to the Over 40 and Still Hot community! I truly mean that. Your commitment to your body, your mind, and your spirit and take it to the next level is what it's all about. The reward is a stronger, sleeker, happier, and of course, sexier YOU!

I know it's not always easy to take time out for yourself. As women, we all seem to be pulled in different directions. Spouses, significant others, kids, jobs, activities as well as friends and family obligations can keep us hopping around. In fact, you might even be wondering how to fit this program into your busy schedule.

It's not because you're busy. That's just a piece of the puzzle. Instead, it's because our physical bodies are changing too. I mean, who hasn't woken up and looked in the mirror and discovered cellulite or back fat where there wasn't any the day before? Not to mention the changes in our skin texture and tone, a few new aches and pains, and the wrinkles that start spreading around eyes, lips, and neck.

However, fitting in a fitness and wellness regime will help you to feel better, look better, sleep better, and deal with all the crazy things you have going on.

Finding new ways to keep yourself motivated, working the muscles in different ways, toning up those trouble spots and mixing up your diet are just some of the things that you'll learn about while reading this eBook. Most importantly, only by merely taking the time to read this eBook, whether you implement everything or not (although I hope that you do!), means that you are receiving the steps to living an active, dynamic life in a way that honors you and your body.

Over 40 and Still Hot is designed to be a total fitness system. It offers challenging and practical exercises that will keep you engaged and motivated so you can get the results that you want. Trust me; you're not alone in having your trouble spots. We all have them. Especially once we start getting around the age of 40, give or take a few years of course. The arms begin to jiggle; the belly pooches, the butt drops, and love handles start to develop. And if you've had any children, well, this tends to speed the process up a little bit. Rest assured, though; it happens to all of us.

Let's face it though. You're getting older. And really, what's wrong with that? Nothing!

Chapter1: What is Menopause?

The first thing I learned was that the weight you gain during menopause doesn't have to be static. I didn't have to suffer it all my life, thank goodness, but before I could even begin to tackle it, I had to thoroughly acquaint myself with what menopause was and the process by which it had allowed fat to settle cozily in my body. Once I understood all the more beautiful details, I would be better prepared to take effective measures against my weight. Apparently, both my eating and exercising regimes had to change. A new era called for a new plan.

Menopause, I learned, typically happens to women between the ages of 45 and 55. A woman's period won't have come for a year, and she now can't have any more children. The transition to menopause is, however, a long one and it begins long before the final period.

For a great many women, the opposite happens. Their periods are not only irregular but when they do come, they are prolonged and heavy, with the final period being the longest and most substantial. The lengthy time between each period is rarely a time of bliss. The uterus may feel stressed, the stomach bloated and cramped, and the breasts heavy and sore. Premenstrual tension is often experienced and can go on for as long as this late waiting period.

Additionally, the woman experiences periodic hot flashes, which last about 30 seconds each time. The hot flashes begin with a feeling of intense heat on the forehead, face, and chest, which soon turns into a sweat which is sometimes cumbersome. Other symptoms may be vaginal dryness, poor sleep patterns, and mood swings. The heart starts to thump vigorously or irregularly. Fatigue sets in. The feelings of discomfort may lead to a woman wanting to rest most of the time, and the result is a more inactive lifestyle and weight gain.

Women experience these menopausal symptoms in varying degrees. They are a natural consequence of aging that all women experience. The transition can last a few years, or go on for more than ten years. It may start in the mid 30's, but it more often begins around the mid 40's.

Although fertility levels dwindle because of lowered estrogen levels, a woman may still conceive during this time. The ovaries are still partly active. This is when uncontrolled weight gain often starts, even if a woman appears to be eating well and exercising regularly. A woman is considered to have reached proper menopause when the period hasn't come for 12 months. The ovaries are no longer functional. She will not conceive after this time.

The hot flashes and other associated conditions may continue far ahead, and additionally, there may be joint, muscle and back pain, as well as heart disease, and the skin is more prone to tears. It's difficult for a woman to control her weight during the transition to menopause and beyond. She may gain an average of 15 lbs. Often she is stressed and irritable. Food seems to be the only relief.

Well, I gained all of 40 lbs during my transitional phase and beyond. Most of this weight was concentrated in the stomach. In my earlier years, when I'd gained weight, I'd done so mainly around the hips, and my figure was more pear-shaped, but now the large is packed primarily around the waist, and I was as round as an apple. I was often tired and fed up, and because of it, my dietary choices were sometimes not the best, but this abdominal fat, I learned, left me more prone to cardiovascular disease and typed II diabetes.

Both were chronic conditions that I wished to avoid at all costs. If left unchecked, I would have a very stressed old age. I had to do something about my weight gain and my shrinking muscle mass here and now. I also spent a lot of time sitting, and the more you sit, it seems, the more muscle you lose, but you gain about the equivalent of the lost muscle mass as body fat. That's because as you lose muscle, the body's ability to use calories slows, as well.

How menopause affects weight loss

Menopause is defined as the cessation of the menstrual process. This natural event happens to ladies aged 40 to 55 years old. Apart from hot flushes and hot flashes, another lousy thing occurs during menopause – weight gain that is hard to shrug off.

Before menopause, your ovarian follicles produce estrogen that plays a significant role in vital life functions, such as skin and vessel maintenance, bone formation and resorption, protein synthesis, coagulation, fluid balance and lung function.

Since menopause halts the ovarian production of estrogen, the body makes up for the lost hormone by prodding the adipose or fat tissues to synthesize the estrogen that the body needs. As such, the organization deposits more and more fatty tissues to continue the development of estrogen. As a result, an older woman usually gain bulges in the breast, buttock and abdominal areas.

Apart from fat-produced estrogen, other mechanisms pave the way for weight gain during menopause. For one, you will experience decreased muscle mass because of a lower metabolic rate and reduced production of thyroid hormones. With reduced muscle mass and a more moderate metabolic rate, lower caloric intake is needed. So your former eating habits which kept you in shape for the longest time can lead to weight gain, even if there is nothing much that has changed in your daily life.

The type of foods you should eat

While you need to cut down on your dietary intake because of menopause and other bodily events, you need to eat several kinds of foods to help with physical functions and daily activities. Here are the foods you should eat daily, as well as the servings that are appropriate for your age, according to the National Institutes of Health:

• Fruits – 1.5 to 2.5 cups

Nuts are rich in vitamins, minerals, and fibers that can help you lose weight. They can also help decrease your chances of succumbing to stroke, heart attack, and other age-related problems. Best of all, fruits are good alternatives for women looking for sweet and healthy foods to end their meals.

• Vegetables – 2 to 3.5 cups

Like fruits, vegetables contain vitamins, minerals, and fibers that can help you shed the excess pounds, apart from protecting your body from diseases and illnesses.

• Grains – 5 to 10 ounces

Grains are miracle foods that can help with weight management. Apart from their effects on weight, grains can also reduce constipation events, as well as your risks of suffering from heart disease.

• Protein-rich foods – 5 to 7 ounces

Protein is a substance that is vital for a lot of bodily processes. It serves as the building blocks of muscles, skin, bones, cartilage, and skin. It is also needed for the synthesis of vitamins, minerals, and enzymes in the body.

• Dairy foods – 3 cups of low-fat or non-fat milk

Dairy foods such as milk and yogurt can improve your bones, therefore reducing your risks of succumbing to osteoporosis. Apart from strengthening your bones, dairy fares can help reduce the development of heart disease, blood pressure and type 2 diabetes mellitus.

• Oils – 5 to 8 teaspoons

There are several kinds of oils. You need to keep in mind that saturated fats can affect your heart health, so make sure to lean towards oil containing monounsaturated and unsaturated fats. Suitable examples of healthy oils include olive oil, flax-seed oil, and nut oils.

• Solid fats and added sugars – Keep the portions small

Good eating habits to adopt

Losing weight is not just about cutting specific food categories in your diet, it is also about incorporating some foods and increasing the intake of some fares to provide your body with the calories it needs. Here are some eating habits that can help you lose weight and live a healthier life as an older woman:

• Drink lots of water.

Senior women usually lose their sense of thirst. Before they know it, they are already checked in the hospital because of dehydration. To prevent the costly medical expenses related to your lack of appetite, make sure to drink water or other liquid beverages whenever you can. Also, add water to your meals by sipping soup every so often.

• Forego fat.

Fat is essential for your body since it provides you energy and helps you synthesize vitamins. But like most foods, too much of a good thing is vile. Too much fat means a lot of calories, which will make you gain weight faster than you can lose it. Keep your waistline trim and your heart healthy by following these recommendations:

1. Choose poultry, meat, and fish without skin.

2. Remove fats from your fish, meat or poultry before cooking them.

3. Make use of low-fat dressing and dairy products.

4. Don't use additional fat when preparing. If you need to, use oils with unsaturated or monounsaturated fats. Cook with non-fat pots and pans.

5. Avoid frying your foods. A healthier

• Eat foods rich in fiber.

Constipation is common in senior women. To prevent this from happening, you need to eat foods rich in fiber, such as fruits, vegetables, seeds, nuts, beans and whole grains.

Fiber is standard in most foods, the way you can make the most out of your intake is to follow these tips:

1. Incorporate lentils, peas and dry beans in your daily meals.

2. Eat fruits and vegetables with their skins on, if possible.

3. Eat fruits instead of drinking fruit juices.

4. Choose whole-grain cereals and bread over traditional products.

Apart from promoting intestinal health, fiber-rich foods can also help lower your blood sugar and cholesterol levels.

• Decrease your salt intake.

Where salt goes, water follows. So if you are fond of salty, cured foods, chances are you will be experiencing hypertensive episodes more often than not. For your age, you need to cut back on your salt intake. According to the National Institutes of Health, salt intake for women 51 years old or older should be 1500 milligrams of sodium – equivalent to 2/3 teaspoon of table sugar.

• Avoid foods with empty calories.

Several foods and beverages are plentiful in 'empty' calories that can make you gain more weight. Keep your weight healthy by avoiding empty calorie foods such as cookies, chips, soda and alcoholic beverages.

• Eat according to your lifestyle.

Do you live an active lifestyle? Or are you sedentary most of the time? Your food intake should be dependent on your activity level. According to USDA, a senior woman who is not physically active should take a limit of 1600 calories, while a lady with a mid-active lifestyle should ingest foods containing 1800 calories every day.

However, if you are very active and immerse in physical activities daily, your caloric intake should range from 2000 to 2200.

The Depletion of the Weight Control Hormones

Menopause prepares the ground for a midlife weight crisis. It causes fluctuations in certain hormones that control issues to do with body weight. The hormones in question include estrogen, progesterone, and testosterone. As these hormones lessen, we desire more and more fat and sugar and turn our backs on foods rich in protein and fiber. Our bodies become prone to fat and water storage. All these factors may contribute to weight gain. The even physical activity we automatically performed declines without us even realizing it. Other menopausal symptoms such as tiredness, poor sleep patterns, and depression contribute to the problem. We don't stand enough or walk around enough.

Estrogen is generated in the ovaries. It controls reproductive issues such as fertility and the menstrual cycle. During the transition to menopause, as a woman's ovaries start to generate a reduced amount of estrogen, her body looks for the lost estrogen outside of the ovaries. Estrogen is also produced in the fat cells, but the fat cells are unable to burn as many calories as muscle cells do.

Decreased estrogen causes a decrease in muscle mass. This means we cannot burn as many calories. This contributes to a slowed metabolism and increased weight gain. Estrogen controls the even distribution of fat in the body, but as estrogen declines, the fat starts to be concentrated around our midriffs.

This is a dangerous place for storing 20 or more pounds of fat; a study has shown. It makes us more prone to cardiovascular disease, diabetes, stroke, heart and kidney disease, insulin resistance, sleep apnea, osteoporosis, high blood pressure, breast cancer and other serious ailments. A sign that a woman's midriff is unhealthily large is when it measures 35 inches or more in circumference.

Diminished estrogen has also been linked to excessive cortisol, which causes increased appetite and therefore fat storage. To make up for the deficit in estrogen, we need to burn more calories through more intense exercise and a better eating plan. Since muscle mass has decreased, we need to use weights to build it up again.

During the meltdown between the ages of 45 and 55, the estrogen is not reduced in one go. It's a gradual wearing off a process that can go on for some years. The duration depends on one's physiology. Reduced estrogen levels give way to hot flashes, vaginal dryness, mood swings, headaches and loss of libido.

Before the menopausal transition, estrogen works with progesterone to help maintain healthy body weight. Progesterone levels begin to reduce earlier than estrogen. A woman is more liable to water retention during menopause. The more water weight she has, the more bloated she is and this reduces the amount of progesterone in her system. This has significant implications for weight gain.

Normal estrogen and progesterone levels in combination will combat the adverse effects of both cortisol and insulin. Left unchecked for extended periods, insulin and cortisol combine to encourage fat storage in the belly and to prevent muscle building up.

Another hormone with similar effects is androgen. The levels of this hormone increase with the advent of menopause. While cortisol and insulin encourage belly fat storage, androgen directs the new body fat straight to the midsection, rather than to the hips where it would typically go.

Another hormone in decline during the menopause transition years is testosterone. The aging process will have already produced a slower metabolism, but depleted amounts of testosterone slow it down even more. The normal function of testosterone is to enable the female body to build lean muscle mass from the calories eaten. The metabolic rate goes up because more calories are being burned by the muscle cells than by the fat cells, but with less testosterone being produced, the number of calories giving way to lean muscle mass declines, leading to a weakened metabolism.

Another weighty problem is insulin resistance. It arises when the body is unable to rid the blood of excess sugar. The more processed food the body takes in, the more strength there is to insulin generated in the bloodstream. The organs don't respond to insulin and the amount of glucose in the blood increases, so all in all, the body has failed to perform its function of ridding the blood of excess sugar. The blood sugar levels are too high, and the inevitable result is weight gain.

However, weight gain at this time is not due only to hormonal imbalances. Our bodies experience increased growth up to the age of about 30, but after that, our physical abilities gradually decline and with this, our skills to work out efficiently, so we burn fewer calories which means depleted muscle mass and weight gain. We find it increasingly difficult to adjust to the changed lifestyle brought by increased age. We are more laid back.

When we retire, for instance, we are no longer tied to a routine. We relax more, socialize more and travel more. We spend lots of time in front of the TV for want of something to do. All in all, our lifestyles become increasingly sedentary. We may feel more tired and depressed, and this adds to the problem. Stress encourages the production of cortisol and reduced estrogen levels, which stimulates a greater appetite and fat storage.

While some women may feel liberated by the coming of menopause, others think bereft by the loss of their fertility. This could lead to binging and a poor diet. As could the emptiness we feel when our children leave home. We may have additional strains like looking after old parents or bereavement. Menopause is undoubtedly a period of tremendous challenge for women.

Losing weight is becoming tougher and tougher after menopause. Many women over 40 have a sedentary lifestyle with not sufficient exercise. Regular exercise is a crucial component to losing weight permanently- however, do you know how much activity is required to lose weight? You might say "the more, the better," and you are right- theoretically. After all, the standard thinking is The more calories you burn, the more weight you lose.

Chapter 2: Health Versus Physical Fitness

Making a Plan

One does not have to be stuck with menopausal weight gain. It is up to us to do what we can to make an active lifestyle and a balanced diet a way of life. Weight loss at this time should be a transforming experience. It's hard work, but the rewards are body and mind wellness.

The early days after I decided to do something about my weight were tough times. I had gained 40 lbs over ten years, and naturally, I was impatient to get it off, but my early efforts were initially marked by lots of fits and starts. When I forced myself to stop, take a deep breath and proceed at a slow and deliberate pace, that was when I started to lose weight.

After this, I was energized and bolstered by every success, however small. Every time I made a significant health decision, I was inspired to do more. My healthy habits were becoming a lifestyle. I wasn't happy to just sit around. I lost about 10 pounds a month. Of course, it's always tempting to go for a size that wasn't made for one's body, such as Size 0, but being Size 0 means being underweight, and being skinny is just as disastrous for the health as being overweight. I planned to go back to my ideal weight of 135 pounds and to introduce much-needed balance into my life.

Losing Weight: Eating Plan

Weight management during menopause rests mainly on controlling what you eat, so my initial focus was on creating a diet plan. First of all, the crash diets had to go. Crash diets require you to cut out nutrient-rich carbohydrates that are essential to good health. They also help to deplete the hormones that control the appetite, so that instead of burning fat, the body burns vital muscle tissue instead. Generally speaking, the crash diets slow the metabolism and make weight gain all the more likely.

I needed something that would sponge up and then get rid of all the excess oils and fats caused by my hormonal deficiencies. I needed to make up for those depleted hormones so I could lose weight. The recipe for weight loss management is clear: lots of fresh fruit, veggies, and whole grains, lots of protein, fiber and water, and exercise at least five days a week for 30 minutes.

The secret to my weight loss, I realized, lay in tweaking my eating plan here and there to make it more relevant to my time and situation, so it could help me maintain my health going forward. I'd eaten a lot of healthy foods in the past, but clearly, what had worked for me when I was 40 no longer applied in my menopausal years, because of my erratic hormones and other aging problems. I had to put the finger on what was not working. Excess insulin is an increasing problem of menopause. It subverts the ordinary course of fat burning. I needed to reduce all the foods that would stop the insulin surge even the supposedly healthy ones such as some fruit and veggies, the whole, on the other hand, increasing those low in starch and natural sugar. That had to be my new weight loss solution. I needed to give my weight issues more focus than I'd done before. One thing about the body as it ages is that it has to be given time to adjust and then to respond when it's ready. My eating habits had to change.

The first month was one of the adjustments and more adjustments. I concentrated on identifying the areas of my diet and my life that needed fixing and making some limited changes. I realized that some of the food I'd previously thought of as healthy wasn't in fact healthy at all. Suddenly, my cupboards and fridge seemed to be overflowing with unhealthy food choices. A revamp was needed.

I'd eaten reasonable quantities of fried, dairy and baked goods, as well as red meats in my earlier years, and I hadn't had any weight gain issues; but there apparently was a problem now. They were contributing to my weight issues. My solution was to cut back gradually on each of these and to begin to replace them with healthy substitutes.

I stopped buying fried food takeaways. They've almost always been deep-fried, and the oil is dripping from them when you buy them.

When you become more health conscious, you become sensitive to such things.

I now preferred to lightly fry my food myself at home with just a dash of healthy oil, like extra virgin olive. I also firmly opted for skinless chicken and turkey. Previously, the skin had been my favorite part of the meat.

Dairy products were my next consideration. We've always been told how the calcium in dairy products is essential for proper teeth and bones, but the problem with these products is that they are also filled with fat, so my solution was to consume dairy products still but to gradually steer myself towards the low fat or fat-free milk and cheeses.

I'd always loved everything white – bread, pasta, rice, and sugar. Like everything else, they hadn't affected my weight before menopause set in, but now, when I needed as many nutrients as I could get, I found from my research that they presented a problem. They had almost no nutritional value because their goodness had been taken out during manufacturing. Consequently, they were easier to digest, and now more than ever, they were spiking my blood sugar levels and making me increasingly hungry.

I now turned to their healthier substitutes, such as brown rice, whole wheat pasta, whole wheat bread, oats, and barley, because they contained the missing fiber and nutrients that provided my body with the energy needed to burn fat. Furthermore, because they are harder to digest, they are absorbed into the bloodstream more slowly, so they slow cravings and hunger pangs. I reduced my intake of salt considerably; sodium leads to water and fat retention. When necessary, I used sea salt as a substitute.

My meals were mainly a collection of veggies, fruit, lean proteins and whole grains. If I went out to eat, I opted for a healthy dinner of salad and either fish or lean meat and rounded this meal off with water and fruit salad, but I chose to have most of my meals at home because restaurant meals are notoriously large, and therefore encourage overeating.

In the past, whenever I felt hungry in between meals, I snacked on potato chips, chocolate bars, and ice-cream; but now I didn't want to spoil my burgeoning eating plan by slotting them in at irregular hours, so I slowly began to replace them with healthy fruit and vegetable snacks. I went for different varieties and colors. My favorites were carrot, cucumber, butternut, celery, and peppers. It became a habit to cut up the fruit and veggies each morning, so they would be on hand whenever I needed them.

I'd never gone in for raw unsalted nuts before, but I acquired a taste for almonds, walnuts, pistachios, cashews and even plain peanuts. I also added seeds to my diet, as well as beans and lentils.

My fruit choices were another area that needed adjustment. I'd eaten a variety of fruits in the past. I'd go for different colors and flavors here, too. I believed that as long as you ate a lot of fruit, you couldn't go wrong. The good thing about nuts is that they are a low-calorie food packed with nutrients and vitamins, but I now learned that some fruits have more significant weight loss benefits than others. They are the ones that are low in natural sugar such as pears, apples, tangerines, strawberries, blackberries and other berry varieties.

Then there are those high in water content, such as watermelon and grapes, which help with hydration. I naturally stocked up on these fruits and found that a general mix of them made for a healthy and tasty snack or after meal dessert. This is not to say that fruits with a high sugar content are a terrible choice. They're OK when eaten in moderation, but when overdone, the fructose within them may contribute to weight gain.

Again, with veggies, some are more potent fat busters than others. I'd always eaten a variety of vegetables, rightly assuming that all plants are healthy, but as with fruit, some have higher slimming value – the green leafy vegetables, in particular. As they digest more slowly into the bloodstream, they enable more fat to be burned, so while continuing to eat a variety of veggies, I increased my intake of the greens. They help rid the body of toxin buildup, which contributes to problems that cause more fat issues such as constipation, stress and bloating. The digestive tract and the liver are more cleansed efficiently. The greens more effectively counter the harmful effects of processed foods like white rice, potatoes, white bread and white flour. There are lots of cheap varieties on the market, from kale and mustard greens to spinach and Bok Choy.

Fruits and veggies, together with whole grains and legumes, have a high fiber content that's important for weight loss. Fiber helps to control insulin and to keep the intestines in top working order. It pumps up the energy and helps you feel full for a prolonged period. The leafy green vegetables possess both fiber and protein. I found that four servings a day of both fruit and veggies helped my weight loss goals.

Veggies and fruit can be hard to preserve. They lose their freshness very quickly, but instead of throwing them out, I found that converting them into smoothies made for a healthy and delicious alternative. I'd eaten veggies before, in smaller quantities than the starch and fatty meat on my plate, but now my dish was dominated by greens. I restricted to rice, potatoes, pasta and lean meat to mere handfuls. Despite the restrictions, there are lots of delicious recipes online to make your eating experiences worthwhile, so long as you stay away from deep frying and opt for healthy cooking styles such as baking, boiling and grilling, and use appropriate oils such as fish oil, avocado oil, and extra-virgin olive oil. There are many right herbal seasonings, too.

I was concerned about losing muscle mass because my weight loss depended on my building up and maintaining my muscle mass, so it was vital for me to get lots of nonfatty protein varieties into my diet. Building up muscle is crucial for anyone seriously wanting to lose weight. It's the number one calorie burner and is key to regulating the metabolism, and the way to building up muscle mass is by eating protein-rich food.

To make up for the depletion of the weight control hormones such as estrogen, progesterone, and testosterone, I consumed lots of seafood because it's rich in omega-3 and omega-6 fatty acids, which help in the breakdown and digestion of food. They help to control your mood and keep you focused on your plan.

More than ever before, I was carefully monitoring what was on my plate, and I was now counting my calories judiciously. I was careful to eat a minimum of 1700 calories a day. It was what I needed to lose around 10 pounds per month. I used advice from the Internet to ensure that I had the right servings of all the food I was eating. I also carefully studied food labels. Health experts say middle-aged women need to provide consumption of 1,650 to 2000 calories a day. That's considered a healthy weight maintenance allowance.

However, counting calories when I went out was a challenge. There's no way of adequately measuring, but the National Institute of Health asserts that protein pieces should be no more than the size of the palm, and starches should be limited to fistfuls.

Consuming different foods from the various food groups took care of my nutritional needs, filled me up and helped me to lose weight because I chose those with the least calories. Daily, I was managing to have 9 ounces of grains, 6 ounces of protein, 2 cups low fat or fat-free dairy products, 2 cups each of fruit and veggies. I had never felt healthier. I looked right, felt lighter and was losing two to three pounds per week.

All in all, I was losing weight at the rate of 10 pounds per month. I was taking in lots of fiber through the grains, fruit, and veggies I was eating, and I was supplementing this intake with nuts and seeds. The texture was slowing the digestive process and staving off the hunger for extended periods. I had enough protein to maintain lean muscle mass and to help stave off weight gain. My protein choices included eggs, fish, lean meats, beans, nuts, and seeds.

The important thing I'd learned from crash diets was not to turn my back entirely on my favorite foods – the ice-creams, the chocolate cakes and the chocolate bars. I found that I still lost weight when I confined myself to a small treat once or twice a week. That gift could be a piece of cake, a 500ml chocolate bar or an ice-cream on a stick. I ate fast foods, at the most, only twice a month. Whatever your food fetish – candy, cookies, chips – moderation is the key factor. You don't have to give it up altogether, but you need to cut back on it. I looked forward to the days of the treatment and was careful not to binge.

By the same principle, while I increased my intake of veggies and fruit, and decreased that of starchy foods and dairy products, I did not drop them altogether, I just ate less of them. I also ate less red meat and confined myself to the lean variety, and while I ate beans and nuts because of their protein content, I was careful to limit my intake to mere handfuls at a time. It seems that these products are also filled with starch or fat.

In the beverages department, I was now drinking as much water as I could comfortably take in. I'd never been a great water drinker, but I did try the recommended eight glasses a day for a while; however, I always felt saturated and heavy the whole day, so I cut down to more manageable levels which I maintain today. I never once felt dehydrated and continued to lose weight. Studies have shown that dehydration helps slow the metabolism and therefore to encourage weight gain.

I also found that water filled me up between meals, and helped me control my cravings. It helped me to digest my food properly and to have regular bowel movements.

I cut out soda completely, and other drinks with excessive amounts of sugar, as well as the so-called diet drinks. Studies have shown that the artificial sugar content in diet drinks makes you fat. It slows the metabolism, leading to cravings and binging on unhealthy foods. It's also been known to cause thyroid problems, which too mess up the metabolism and the body's ability to handle and process foods.

I'd never been a great alcohol drinker, and I wanted to keep it that way. I avoided it completely. The thing about alcohol is that it has a high calorie and sugar content, and can add to weight problems. Alcohol encourages cravings for more alcohol, while caffeine related drinks cause erratic energy and mood levels, and are best avoided.

In the drinks department, I opted for water and a variety of delicious natural beverages that enhanced, rather than spoiled, my eating plan. I found green tea particularly satisfying. It has properties that speed up the metabolism and therefore help you to lose excess weight. These features also reduce the process by which fat is taken into the body, and this results in low weight and cholesterol levels; and like water, it keeps the appetite at bay in-between meals. It slows down the entry of fat in the body when drunk before meals.

I found Ginseng Tea to be another excellent fat buster. It revs up the energy and allows us to be active for more extended periods during the day. It also normalizes blood sugar levels, and in this way, it helps carbohydrates from being converted into fat. The metabolism is boosted, and fat is burned more quickly.

Coconut water has similar effects. It speeds up the metabolism and helps to burn fat quickly, and it also has low calorie and sugar levels. I found it to be a brilliant hydrant as well, but read the label. It has a naturally sweet flavor of its own. Don't buy coconut waters with added sugar.

Rather than having three square meals, I found I lost more weight when I had three small meals, with snacks in between to stave off hunger.

Studies have shown that cutting the amount on your plate but increasing the number of times you eat helps your metabolism to work as it should.

Sample Meal Plan

Breakfast

One hard-boiled egg, 1 cup oatmeal with fat-free milk.

First Snack

A handful of nuts/seeds

Half a cup of fruit

Lunch

Grilled fish, a handful of brown rice and 1 cup spinach, fruit salad

Second Snack

Half a bowl of fruit

A handful of nuts/sees

Dinner

Grilled chicken, mixed green salad, mixed fruit salad

A valuable lesson in my menopausal weight loss journey was that healthy eating did not necessarily translate into fat loss. You can eliminate all processed foods, get as close to nature as possible in your eating habits, eat lots of healthy proteins cooked in low-fat oils, and still, you will not notice any difference in weight. How much do you have on your plate? Portion size is important. There is no difference between 1 cup of white rice and 1 cup of brown rice in weight loss matters. The brown rice will, of course, offer much more fiber which is essential for weight loss, but eating lots of it doesn't cause faster weight loss. You have to watch your portion size, whatever the healthy food, and whether it's fat-free, fiber-rich, or protein-rich. You can't eat these healthy foods in excess. Just a fistful of the brown rice is sufficient, for instance.

You have to learn to get the better of ghrelin, the hunger hormone if you're to lose weight efficiently. Make it a point to eat breakfast, and at the same time each day. Always ensure that it's the main meal of the day because it will serve to energize you for the remainder of the day. It will help to regulate the rest of your meals, so in effect, breakfast helps to control ghrelin, the hunger hormone and helps you reach your weight loss goals for the day.

Don't miss any of your meals or snack times. To regulate ghrelin, you would have to eat every three hours or so. Ensure that within a day, you have eaten food from all the leading food groups, too – fruit and veggies, protein-rich, and fiber-rich food groups, and ensure you have the right mix to stave off hunger and cravings and acquire energy to burn calories.

Carbohydrates such as brown rice or lentils, sweet potatoes, grains, and fruit will reduce the ghrelin, increase brain power and keep cravings at bay. You also get enough protein to stop the loss of muscle mass and invigorate your metabolism. Eat every morsel of food deliberately, staying in the moment and enjoying every bit of it so you can have a satisfying feeling of fullness at the end. Give your eating process your full attention. Sit somewhere quiet where there are no distractions. In time, you will learn to identify when you are starving and need to eat and how much actually to eat before you get full. Drinking water will also help stave off your hunger and keep you hydrated.

With this kind of plan, you don't need limiting diet plans that you can't sustain. They may even reorder your body for you. While slowing your metabolic rate and boosting ghrelin, the hunger hormone, they will lower your level of leptin, the hormone related to fullness. This makes it doubly difficult for you to lose weight. The weight loss plan described here boosts your digestive process and staves off hunger, enabling you to eat less but still stay full for longer.

Losing Weight: Exercise Plan

Exercise helps to complete the weight loss program. It's best to get advice from the doctor, first, before beginning any severe activities.

If suffering from a particular injury or painful problem, you may not be able to do specific tasks. As with your eating plan, you have to change up your workouts.

What worked in the past may not necessarily work now. It's a different era. Your exercises will be slower, but more applicable to your menopausal status. Moderate physical activity is what's recommended. You will not be gasping for breath, just breathing more quickly, and you will burn at least three calories every minute. As your base exercise, you should do cardio workouts that you enjoy and switch them up regularly to stay interested. If you get on your elliptical machine every day against your will, you will quickly develop an aversion to it, so avoid it if it's not for you. You could try getting a family member or friend to embark on this exercise program with you, but your experience will always be a personal one and is all about hands-on involvement.

There are so many exercises to choose from – brisk walking, cycling, swimming, dancing, and aerobics being a few popular ones. These practices are good for the vast muscles, and they contribute to weight loss, but they should be done at a moderate pace. I combined walking with aerobics. I started slow, but gradually built up to five 30-minute aerobic sessions a day and daily 20-minute walks, but I didn't stop there.

I added another dimension to my exercise program – weightlifting. It proved crucial to my weight loss regime. It helped me to build muscle mass and to burn fat, therefore, faster than I would have with cardio alone.

An eating plan by itself is insufficient. It doesn't raise the metabolism high enough. Only the building of lean muscle will do that, and this happens through strength training. It's not necessary to sign up for a gym or invest in expensive equipment. Various cheap hand weights and other supporting material are available in sports shops or online.

One of the main reasons why we lose muscle mass, leading to a lowered metabolism and then weight gain, is that our lives are too sedentary. It's all about sitting – at the computer, the TV, and the work desk. It starts when we're younger and develops into a habit we can't break when we're older.

That applied to me in many ways. The 20-minute periods of exercise were virtually the only physical exertion I had allowed myself previously. I had sat around a lot of the time. Then I couldn't understand why my body stayed flabby and why I was getting rounder.

A sound exercise plan I found, is part of an overall active lifestyle. More calories are burned standing than sitting, studies have found. Sitting lowers the metabolic process considerably, leading to secure fat storage. If you have a sedentary type of job, interject periods of standing into your daily routine. You could stand and move around every 30 minutes. If your situation permits it, you could do some of your work on the computer while holding.

My exercise program had a lot of fits and starts, but every time I felt discouraged, I got myself back up again by reminding myself of why I was doing it. I told myself, too, that my excess weight was playing havoc with my self-esteem and could lead to a myriad of chronic ailments like heart disease and diabetes if I gave up. That proved motivation enough and I'd be energized again.

I was determined that my workouts should be useful. Throwing weights into the mix was crucial because it helped me to exercise more muscles and burn more calories. I tried some exercises and was careful to avoid those that weighed down my knees and those that worked only one muscle group, such as leg curls and leg extensions. I found that lifting and squatting exercises helped to strengthen my body and to burn many calories while building up my core strength and stabilizing my muscles. \

After learning the basics of the tasks, I turned to raising the intensity level slightly, because of the more intense the activities, the more the calories I burned. This was crucial to increased weight loss. Strength training has impressive health benefits for menopausal women and those that are older, who are also subject to osteoporosis. With strength training, bone density is enhanced, and the risks of colon cancer and cardiovascular disease are reduced. Hand weights strengthen the body and improve posture, and enhance the back against potential injury. Start with light hand weights and restrict the repetitions to 8, increasing them little by little till you get to 12 reps.

Studies have shown that one can lose 4 pounds of weight in 10 weeks from merely doing strength exercise, and I had managed to lose 40 pounds in four months by combining these strength exercises with a healthful eating plan. The practices are highly beneficial for menopausal women if all the muscle groups are dealt with in a single training session.

In both the weight and cardio exercises, I was careful not to push myself harder than was safe for my body. I refrained from the high impact exercises. These include throwing and jumping and are not recommended for women past 50. They are injurious to the bones and ligaments. It's safer to do exercises that place the least pressure on the joints.

High-intensity cardio was also out of the question for someone of my age. I tried it out and found that, although I could push myself for shorter spells, it left me breathing so hard I couldn't talk. The moderate intensity exercise level was just right for me, while the low-intensity level I kept for my warm-ups and cooldowns. The thing about a combined exercise program is that it helps keep you active and therefore prevents weight gain.

Studies have shown that older persons increasingly need more exercise to lose weight, so I had my five 30-minute cardio sessions, which I would follow up each day with a brisk 20-minute walk, and then I had two 30-minute weight training sessions slotted in during the week. This was a comprehensive program, and I believed it would help me achieve my weight loss goals, but what is quantity without quality? It doesn't translate into much. I endeavored to make my exercises as active as possible and get the highest benefit potential in the time I'd set aside. Exercising at a gym with others was a bonus. Everyone kept commenting on my continued transformation. It buoyed me.

A few weeks into the first month of my new lifestyle plan, I was already feeling on top of the world. I had managed to lose 5 pounds from my combined eating and exercise programs. I looked better and was moving better. Two-thirds of my time had been spent sitting in front of the TV and the computer, but now I was paying only a third of my time there. The rest of the time I was exercising, and doing housework and gardening.

My cardio exercises were not confined solely to aerobics. When I found myself getting bored, I would switch to the elliptical machine or dancing. Anyone can come up with a suitable program. Cycling, swimming and jogging and playing tennis are equally valid. It's all about preference. If you're out walking your dog, you can let the dog set the pace and see if you can keep up. It's good exercise as long as you don't tire yourself.

Exercise helps you do something about your hormonal deficiency. Short, intense exercise spells can also promote the increase of growth hormones like testosterone and cortisol, which work together to get rid of fat and maintain muscle mass. That's why short, intense exercise is better for weight loss during menopause.

Long exercise spells affect the hormones differently. They raise the levels of cortisol, but without generating a corresponding balance in the growth hormones, so cortisol's adverse effects become more pronounced. This does not help weight loss matters during menopause, so the shorter types of exercise appear to be more beneficial.

One way to efficiently control and lower cortisol is through relaxation techniques such as meditation and massage and sauntering while practicing deep breathing or only walking at a relaxing place. This, together with a diet that reduces insulin, can help you make tremendous strides in your weight loss program. Estrogen and progesterone, which would have reduced the insulin and its effects, are lacking.

I found it beneficial to keep a diary where I recorded my meals and workouts to help me follow my progress, hold myself accountable and amend anything that wasn't working for me. If weight gain just seems to happen again, adjust your eating plan and rev up your exercises, or find out if there's an area of your life that's responsible for the weight gain. Make notes of whatever you're eating at a particular time and how you feel about it. This helps with the adjustments you think you have to make. Have your journal with you at all times so you can quickly check what you are doing right or wrong. It will also contain notes about steps you are taking to stay active outside of your eating and fitness regime.

If you can't work out regularly, or feel stressed or fretful at any stage, find other ways to occupy yourself, such as learning a new hobby, craft, or language. Join a yoga class, take up reading, or train a puppy and take it for daily walks. Ignore the elevator and take the stairs. Walk to colleagues' offices for consultations, instead of calling them on the phone or sending e-mails. Have meetings with colleagues in places where you're forced to stand. Walk fast as often as possible.

Training a puppy can be enormously rewarding. You are teaching the puppy in the ways of the world, and it keeps your mind concentrated on the task. You do not have time to fret about your weight loss problems, and it takes your account off eating. You can adapt your routine to the puppies. Fitness plans are more accessible to achieve when you have a method so that you would have a schedule for your puppy's entire life, such as sleep time, mealtime, playtime and toilet time. This adds direction to your life. Each time you train your puppy in new habits, you are boosting your program.

Just don't become sedentary again. You don't want to let depression interfere with the excellent work you've done on your body and the new self-confidence that stemmed from the process. Maintaining a positive attitude is essential. Relaxation releases any tension that may have built up from your first regime. It keeps you on track during your menopausal weight loss journey. Learn deep breathing exercises to aid in relaxing the muscles. Rest when you need to. Be sure to get at least 7 hours of sleep each night.

Relaxation activities release serotonin and endorphins, which make us happier and more settled. You might want to do meditation for about 10 minutes following an exercise routine. This will give you a greater sense of wellness. Focus on your breathing. Take a deep inward breath, pushing your stomach forward. Hold the movement. Then let out the air slowly through your nose, pushing your stomach in as far as possible. Let your thoughts pass freely in and out of your head without denying or attaching yourself to any of them. This way, you demystify and accept them more, and eventually find solutions to whatever is troubling you. Your cravings will also filter in and out, and you will similarly find ways around them. The more you practice, the more relaxed you become. You let go of problems that are in the way, that doesn't serve you. You learn inner peace and focus.

Chapter3:Weight Management in Women over 40

Some things just get more comfortable with age. Driving a car, playing a musical instrument or sinking a 40-foot putt. Unfortunately, so does gaining weight.

Women over 40 are particularly concerned about their weight. Physical appearance, linked with poor self-esteem can wreak havoc with women who are still at the peak of their earning capacities. Competing with younger, often more attractive women can exacerbate a problem women have known about for years: gaining weight is almost an inevitable part of growing older.

And, obesity is an equal opportunity epidemic. Weight gain affects just as many women as men over the age of 25, with obesity rates skyrocketing in those over 40. But, how did we get so fat?

Cave-dwelling women never worried about their weight. While the menfolk were outside chasing down dinner, they remained inside crushing nuts and berries, tanning hides and vacuuming the dirt floor. In short, women stayed active.

It's only been during the past 20 years that women have begun watching their waistlines expand. Between ages 25 to 44, women can expect their basal metabolic rates (the body's innate idling speed) to decline as much as three percent per decade.

At 20 years of age, basal metabolic rates account for up to 70 percent of a woman's total energy expenditure, declining 150 calories a day, per decade. That translates to as much 1.5 extra pounds a year—without making any changes to lifestyle.

A meaningful debate regarding age- and gender-related fitness standards has resulted in two measures: health fitness and physical fitness. The health fitness standards are based on minimum fitness values for disease prevention and health. For a person to attain the health and fitness standards requires only moderate physical activity. For example, a 2-mile walk in less than 30 minutes, five or six times per week, seems to be sufficient to achieve the health-fitness standards for cardiorespiratory endurance.

Significant health benefits can be reaped with such program, although fitness improvements are not as notable.

These benefits include a reduction in blood lipids, lower blood pressure, stress release, less risk for diabetes, and more economic risk for chronic diseases and premature mortality.

More specifically, improvements in the metabolic profile (measured by insulin sensitivity, glucose tolerance, and improved cholesterol levels) can be notable despite little or no weight loss or increase in aerobic capacity. Metabolic fitness can be attained through an active lifestyle and moderate-intensity physical activity.

A Primer on Weight Loss: Why it can Seem So Hard

For many women, the journey to obesity begins right after college graduation. Along with higher annual salaries, come time-saving perks and services. Things women used to take care of themselves are added to a long list for the housekeeper or babysitter. With each promotion, comes more responsibility, emotional stress, less leisure time and a parking place close to the office. As families and schedules grow, there's less time to devote to exercise and taking care of themselves. When they do, it's usually an hour massage with a glass of pinot noir instead of a vigorous hike outdoors in the fresh air. At the first inkling of extra weight, they'll inevitably skip lunch throwing their blood glucose levels into a tailspin. By the time dinner arrives, they're ravenous and end up eating twice as much as they usually would. Sound familiar?

There's no secret to losing weight over 50. It begins with a simple equation: calories in equal calories out. In short, whenever there's a gain or loss on either side, you gain or lose weight. Unfortunately, it's not that simple. Some additional factors are waiting to play havoc with women trying to lose weight; more specifically, fat mass.

That means over 75 percent of a woman's whole body weight should be fat-free, lean tissue. You can have your fat and fat-free mass measured (called body composition testing) at a doctor's office, physical therapy clinic or local colleges and universities that have active physical education programs. You can also Google "body composition" for more information about where you can get tested.

The most relevant examples of fat-free tissue are muscle, skin, bones, body fluids and connective tissue. The fat-free mass is metabolically active, meaning that it burns calories, whether you're active or not. On the other hand, fat mass is used for energy storage; it's only along for the ride. All of us are born with a relatively static number of fat cells that peaks around adolescence. Lean women have between 20 to 27 billion fat cells, while obese women might have between 75 to 300 billion fat cells. Comparing two women of the same weight, one might be considered overweight because more than 25 percent of her total body weight is obese, while the other is normal.

Because fat-free tissue is metabolically active, building or maintaining it should always be at the center of any weight loss program. If it's not, you'll never succeed in permanently losing weight.

As it turns out, where you store body fat is also essential. Physiologists have identified two distinct body types that describe how men and women store fat. Many women have gynoid body types. Frequently called "pear-shaped," gynoid women tend to store the majority of body fat on their hips and thighs toward the back of their bodies. Android, or "apple-shaped" women tend to store most of their body fat around their waist, towards the front. Most men have android body types. Research has shown that men and women who are overweight with android body types have a higher risk for heart disease compared to gynoid body types.

As a woman approaches menopause (usually in her late 40s to early 50s), she begins to experience changes in hormone levels; individually, estrogen, testosterone, leptin, and cortisol. When estrogen is at normal levels, it helps her maintain a healthy weight by increasing insulin, one of the primary hormones responsible for healthy glucose metabolism. During menopause, estrogen levels drop, causing lower metabolic rates. Low estrogen levels also cause the body to process blood sugar less efficiently, making it more difficult to lose weight. Lab studies have shown that lower estrogen levels in animals cause them to eat more and exercise less.

When estrogen levels rise, the pancreas fails to produce adequate amounts of insulin, and the cells of the body become insulin resistant, raising blood glucose levels, much like a person with diabetes. To normalize blood glucose levels, the body begins storing the excess glucose as fat, increasing the size of the fat cells. Sometimes as much as four times their average size. When fat cells around the hip and thighs grow, it can stress the cell walls, causing unsightly cellulite. Nothing short of weight loss can make a difference.

High protein, low fiber diets consisting of large amounts of meat can drive up estrogen levels through xeno-estrogens. Xeno-estrogens are toxins that act like additional estrogen. They're found in many meat products, steroids, and antibiotics. Women may unknowingly ingest xeno-estrogens through herbicides, pesticides and synthetic hormones in cosmetics, lipstick, processed foods and prescription drugs. Xeno-estrogens can overload normal testosterone levels, degrading healthy hormone balance.

Leptin is a frequently occurring hormone that is responsible for telling the brain when you're satiated and have had enough to eat. Diets containing high levels of fructose (a pure sugar found in fruits and fruit juices) convert extra calories into fat, depositing it in the liver and fat cells. Because fat cells monitor leptin levels in the body, leptin levels increase, eventually causing the body to become resistant to it. The brain fails to sense leptin, missing the opportunity to signal the mind that the stomach is full. The result: increased calories and weight gain.

Cortisol, often called the stress hormone, helps the body convert blood sugar into fat. When cortisol levels are high (during fasting, starvation of emotional stress), it throws the body into survival mode, helping it to store fuel for times when food is scarce. You may not be starving, but your body doesn't know the difference. It's programmed to react the same way today as it has for thousands of years. Excessive coffee intake can also increase cortisol levels, so it's a good idea to limit caffeine intake when you're watching your weight.

Everyday food chemicals, while not technically hormones, can act as toxins in the body and impede weight loss. A survey by the Center for Disease Control found that over 93 percent of the American population had measurable amounts of Bisphenol A (BPA), a chemical commonly found in canned foods and plastic containers. BPA interferes with estrogen, thyroid and androgen hormones, impeding their production and metabolism.

Diet and Exercise Solutions: How to Achieve the New You

The first step toward becoming the new you begins with a visit to your doctor's office for a complete physical examination. It's important to rule out underlying causes of weight gain; especially if it's been a while since your last inspection. During the physical exam, your doctor will measure your body mass index (BMI), as well as your vital statistics. They'll also conduct routine blood chemistry analyses that rule out predispositions for heart disease and diabetes, and check hormone levels that might hamper your weight loss efforts. Abnormal hormone levels observed in hypothyroidism can exist for years, lurking under the surface without exhibiting symptoms.

Abnormal blood chemistry levels for cholesterol, glucose and HDL cholesterol could also affect the recommendations your doctor makes for physical activity. Women over 50 should be given a clean bill of health before starting any vigorous exercise programs, especially if they have risk factors for heart disease like high blood pressure, high cholesterol, family history of heart disease, cigarette smoking or diabetes.

Each pound of body fat stores the equivalent of 3500 calories. So, if you're planning to lose 2 lbs. A week that means you'll need to either restrict or expend 7000 calories a week. The best approach is by doing both: plan on limiting 3500 calories by making dietary adjustments, while consuming 3500 calories through regular exercise. That may sound like a lot, but dividing 7000 calories a day by seven days is only 1000 calories a day. To reach your goal, you'll need to restrict 500 calories a day, while expending 500 through exercise. That's equivalent to skipping a Big Mac (without the fries) and taking a brisk walk during your lunch break.

Women over 40 are likely to be firmly entrenched in some negative behaviors, activities, and responsibilities that make losing weight particularly challenging. You may want to look for "shortcuts." Don't be tempted. Your weight loss efforts should be your priority. At times, it might seem impossible, but people do it all the time. Sister Madonna Buder, age 80, has completed 36 Ironman events. At 76, she became the first woman to complete the Hawaiian Ironman: a 1.2-mile swim, followed by a 112-mile bike ride and a 26.2-mile marathon. You can do it.

The Role of Exercise in Weight Loss

At the core of all weight loss programs, is physical activity; especially if you're over 50. As we age, the body loses valuable lean tissue, primarily in the form of bone, muscle, and connective tissue. The results include slower metabolism, fragile bones, loss of balance, more health-threatening falls and increased chances of injury. The antidote to aging is remaining physically active.

Even if you've exercised in the past, it's always a good idea, to begin with, a visit to your doctor. Unless you have risk factors for heart disease or other extenuating circumstances that might impact your ability to exercise, there's no reason why you shouldn't be able to begin today.

Aerobic activity is any activity that uses large muscle groups, allow you to control the exercise intensity and can be sustained for a brief for extended periods of time. Suitable examples of aerobic activity are walking, running, swimming, rowing and hiking. The minimum aerobic requirements for maintaining health include:

Exercising most days of the week, for a total of *150 minutes per week*

Exercising at intensities of *60 – 90 percent of your relative heart rate reserve*. Another way to estimate proper exercise intensity is using the talk test. Walk briskly enough to break a sweat, but can still carry on a conversation with a friend

Exercise at least 30 minutes per session*; more if you can*

In the beginning, finding 30 minutes a day to exercise may be challenging. There's nothing to say that you have to do all 30 minutes at once. Research has shown that people who apply 150 minutes a day, even if it is divided into two or three sessions, receive the same benefits as those who continually use for 30 minutes. If you have significant weight to lose, you'll probably need to use more than 30 minutes a day; possibly as much as 60 to 180 minutes. More on this later.

To realize benefits from exercise and ensure that you're exercising enough to make an impact in your weight loss program, you'll need to exercise vigorously. The easiest way to ensure that you're exercising hard enough (but not too hard) is by measuring your pulse.

Many people ask, "Why is it so important to exercise at a prescribed intensity? Isn't just making an effort good enough?" The answer is yes and no. While any attempt to exercise is indeed better than nothing, exercise frequency, and intensity is particularly important for weight loss. In essence, you're training your body's resting metabolic rate to idle at a faster speed; even after you leave the gym. The higher the exercise intensity, the longer your body will continue idling at a more top rate—which means burning a more significant number of calories throughout the entire day. Even while you're asleep. By exercising every day at the proper intensity, you are raising your body's resting metabolic rate, burning more total calories.

Once you've started, increase your exercise duration slowly; no more than 10-20 percent every two weeks. Many women get so excited with the results they see after a few weeks, they rapidly increase exercise duration, causing debilitating injuries. Go slow. Stay consistent.

Many older women are intimidated by exercise and have specific concerns; mainly how they'll be perceived by others, their physical appearance, their risk of injury. Here are a few things to keep in mind for building a life-long exercise program:

Begin slowly, using activities you know you can do. Unless you are extremely overweight or have orthopedic concerns, walking is often a great place to start. It's an activity you've done all your life, requires very little in the way of specialized equipment, can be done anywhere (even while you're on vacation) and can include family and friends.

Buy a pair of quality walking shoes. Even if you're walking during lunchtime at work, walking will be more enjoyable and comfortable if you use a good quality pair of walking or running shoes.

Use white athletic socks that are a blend of cotton and polyester fabric that wick moisture away from your feet. Wash them frequently and throw them away when they become worn.

Take good care of your feet; especially if you have diabetes. Simple blisters can quickly get infected, becoming debilitating (even life-threatening) injuries, derailing your best efforts to stay active.

If you have lower extremity injuries or are extremely overweight, try non-weight bearing activities like biking, swimming or using an elliptical trainer. Stationary rowing machines are another excellent alternative to the home. Many fitness centers offer water aerobics: classes that are conducted in the shallow end of a swimming pool. Water aerobics provides all the benefits of standard, weight-bearing exercise while supporting the weight of your body. The resistance of the water helps to strengthen abdominal and leg muscles while you exercise.

If you're self-conscience about your appearance, you might want to skip the gym membership in the beginning. Walk outside. If the weather is inclement, see if you can find a large shopping mall. Many malls conduct supervised, morning walking programs for seniors.

Find ways to integrate physical activity into your day. Avoid driving when you can walk. Park further away from the office and use the stairs instead of elevators whenever possible.

Make exercise a regular part of your day. After you establish new, healthy habits, you'll miss practice when you can't schedule it.

Buy a pedometer to help monitor your progress. You can download iPhone and Android pedometer apps like Pedometer++ from the iTunes store. Fitness experts recommend 10,000 steps a day as a reasonable goal. Use it to keep track of how many levels you log throughout the day.

Reward yourself with non-food rewards when you hit significant milestones. Buy yourself a new pair of exercise pants the first time you walk a continuous mile.

Resistance Training in Women Over 40

Once you've established a sound aerobic exercise program, there's still a little more work to do; but not that much. Research has shown that middle-aged men and women who include at least two days a week of resistance training, have more success at losing weight and keeping it off. Women who participate in deficient calorie diets (800 calories/day) often suffer muscle tissue; the tissue they're trying to preserve. Furthermore, the weight they do lose usually returns within six months.

While eating a healthy diet adds structure to your caloric intake and energy balance, resistance training targets the tissues that expend most of your energy: the muscles. It can mean the difference between looking lean and healthy, versus emaciated and gaunt. Maintaining muscle tissue is especially important in older women. As women age, they lose muscle, bone, and connective tissue. There is also evidence that middle-aged adults begin to lose their visual acuity and balance. As a teen, single trips and falls are nothing to be concerned about. As you age, recovering balance is more difficult and can result in serious injuries. According to the Center for Disease Control, more than 250,000 older adults fracture their hips each year. More than three-quarters are women. Resistance training two days a week can help prevent that.

There are two types of resistance training favorite with older women: gravity training and conventional resistance training (often called weight training). If you've never spent time maintaining and developing your muscles, gravity training may be the best way to start. With gravity training, you use the weight of your body against the pull of gravity to develop strength. Suitable examples of gravity training are sit-ups, push-ups, pull-ups, and heel-lifts. You can control the amount of weight you use by modifying exercise posture. Older women may want to start by using the adjusted push-up position, by supporting your weight between your hands and knees. Three sets of ten modified push-ups is a good beginning goal. As you push up, be sure to keep your back straight and look forward instead of down. Once you can quickly complete three sets of modified push-ups, graduate to the standard push-up position: balancing on your toes.

There are dozens of excellent gravity-based exercises you can do anywhere: at home and in the gym. Even in your hotel room. Check with a certified exercise trainer to show you how to perform a complete gravity-based routine for your entire body safely.

Once you've mastered gravity-based resistance training, you'll be ready to graduate to standard weight training. Most YWCAs and fitness facilities have a variety of free weights and machines to help you accomplish your goals. In the beginning, many older women prefer to use tools because they stabilize major muscle groups, helping you achieve a better quality workout. Each device has simple diagrams, explaining the purpose of the engine and how to properly use it. Begin conservatively by choosing a weight that allows you to complete three sets of 10 to 15 repetitions. Look for a machine that exercises the opposing muscle group and uses that next. For instance, after finishing several sets of exercise for the biceps, look for a tool that applies the triceps. Most well-designed fitness centers position opposing devices next to each other to expedite training.

Many women use machines exclusively. They're easy to use and provide high-quality workouts without depending on exercise partners. However, you may want to add or alternate free weights into your program. Free weights provide more concentrated workouts because you work not only the primary muscle groups but the smaller, stabilizing muscle groups as well. Even though the same principles of gravity-based and weight machines apply to free weights, you'll probably notice that you use slightly less weight. It's also a good idea to exercise with a workout partner. Workout partners can monitor your posture, balance and exercise technique and are available should you need help. Regardless of what type of resistance training you choose, be sure to schedule several orientation sessions with a certified exercise trainer to make sure you're performing the exercises correctly to avoid injury.

Psychological and Other Barriers to Weight Loss

Even with the best intent and preparation, losing weight after 50 can be challenging for women. Unlike their younger counterparts, women over 50 have to address some unique challenges before successfully reaching their goal. The good news is that most of them are easy to solve and come slowly with time.

Women over 50 who have never exercised before the need to learn new approaches for integrating physical activity into their lifestyle; both physical and psychological. Often, finding as little as 10 minutes a day can be a daunting dilemma. It makes no difference when you exercise. Walking at lunchtime is just as valid as walking early in the morning or after work. Whatever works for you is the best choice. It's important, though, to try to exercise at the same time, seven days a week. Research has shown that women who use at the same time of day are more likely to make it a permanent part of their life. Many women opt to apply first thing in the morning before their schedules start competing with other responsibilities. On the other hand, walking at lunch or after work can be useful for reducing stress and can be a great antidote to snacking in between meals. Choose what works best for you.

Many women have never exercised because they think it's boring or has never been taught how. If that sounds like you, look into all of the options you have at your disposal: groups, gyms, water-aerobic classes, cycling clubs or outdoor hiking clubs. You're bound to find something you enjoy. Try mixing it up. Nothing says you have to do the same type of exercise every day. Keep in interesting.

Thankfully, the 1980s are gone. The days when women convinced themselves that to exercise they needed to wear the latest Spandex tights and leg warmers. Today, regular exercisers wear whatever is the most comfortable and functional. Older women may want to opt for looser clothing until they feel less self-conscience. Wear whatever makes you the most comfortable.

For people who begin their workday early in the morning, exercising after work may be the only option. But, what do you do when you're just too tired to exercise? The most important thing is to set realistic goals and be easy on yourself. You won't be exhausted every day. Adjust your exercise routines according to your energy levels. Often, just making a start is enough to reclaim your energy level. But above all, avoid flopping on the couch with a bag of Doritos when you get home from work.

Let me dispel one other myth: there is no such thing as "spot reducing." Women over 50 often begin exercising to take care of one, specific area like the back of their arms or to reduce cellulite on their hips. Whether you have 5 or 50 pounds to lose, caloric expenditure happens throughout your entire body—attacking all of your fat cells.

Probably the biggest obstacle to maintaining a regular diet and exercise routine will be yourself. You're up against years of excuses and bad experiences, so begin slowly and take one day at a time. Most women who are successful with their weight loss program have help; either from outside resources or family and friends. Before beginning any weight loss program, tell everyone you know what you're about to do. They'll be there to offer support and resistance when you feel like giving up. If you have doubts about adhering to your new program, enrolling in a weight loss group may be the best move you'll ever make. Research has shown that women have far higher success rates when working together, as opposed to depending solely on themselves.

Chances are, you have a lifetime of extra weight to lose and even more bad habits. Don't let it overwhelm you. Start slowly, stay consistent. You'll be amazed at what you can accomplish.

Weight loss tips for mature women

Since mature women have different bodily events that make weight loss harder, there are 'special tips' for these ladies. If you want to live a healthier and longer life for your kids and grandkids, then here are weight loss tips that can help you drop the excess weight even at your age:

1. Cut down on your fat and sugar intake.

You probably had heard about this when you were still young. It holds true even if you are 50, 60 or 70 years old! This does not mean you should eliminate fat entirely from your diet; you just have to cut foods rich in saturated fat from your diet.

For example, instead of consuming hamburger and fries for lunch, the better alternative is broiled chicken breast and vegetables. When cooking food, make sure to use canola or sunflower oil instead of the usual lard.

Apart from fats, eliminating sugar consumption at your age is another measure that can help you lose weight. Not only will it help you drop some pounds, but it is also especially beneficial if you suffer from diabetes mellitus. Avoid cakes and eat healthier sweets instead, such as fruits. Consume brown rice and whole-wheat bread

instead of its traditional contemporaries. Use Splenda, Sweet N'
Low or other more vigorous forms of sweeteners for your coffee or
tea.

2. Consume calcium-rich foods.

Calcium is known to help older women lose weight. Apart from this,
it also improves the bone health of the individual. As a senior
woman, you are at risk of suffering from osteoporosis, hip fractures
and other events resulting from calcium deficiency. You can prevent
this – and lose weight along the way – by ingesting high-calcium
fares such as milk, dark leafy greens, fortified soy products,
almonds, canned fish, to name a few.

3. Spice up your life.

You might think of this as a boon but adding some spices to your
food can help you lose weight. Some spices can help rev up your
metabolism, therefore enabling you to lose more weight. For tastier
meals that can help you shed the excess pounds, make sure to use
cinnamon, horseradish, and onion in your meals.

4. Make a move.

Even if you are old, it doesn't mean that you should not perform
exercises. Not only will these workouts help you lose weight, but
they can also help you live a better life. According to the USDA, a

minimum of 10 minutes of exercise every day is okay, as long as you perform 150 minutes' worth of workouts every week.

You don't necessarily have to push your body to the limit with crippling workouts. Exercises such as brisk walking, running, swimming and jogging with friends can help you lose weight and have a fun time all at the same time.

5. Lift weights.

An excellent accompaniment to cardiovascular exercises is weightlifting, as this can help you tone your muscles and eliminate the sagging, flabby skin on your arms, thighs, and stomach. Like exercises, you don't have to punish yourself with 25-pound weights. Start off with 2-pound weights and gradually go up as you build resistance.

6. Drink lots of water.

Water keeps you hydrated; your skin is soft and supple. Apart from these benefits, water can help you lose weight since it makes you feel full, therefore eliminating your tendency to snack fatty and sugary foods in between meals.

7. Sleep well.

Sleep does not only rejuvenate your mind and your body, but it can also help you lose weight. Studies show that lack of sleep can lead to more eating binges and other bodily changes that make weight loss a problematic activity to carry out.

Chapter4: How to sleep to lose weight now

Sleep is something that gets lost in just about every discussion about fat, weight loss, fat loss and body composition.

We all have some understanding that we should be eating better and moving more, but few people understand the enormous impact that sleep has on weight loss. Researchers have found that those who logged 7 to 9 hours a night had healthier body weights than those who slept less.

I remember once being told that you can't eat and exercise your way out of poor sleeping habits. It's so true. Over the years I have had many clients whose exercise and eating habits have been perfect but struggle to lose weight because of poor or inadequate sleep.

Did you know that by going without enough sleep for just two nights is detrimental?

Hopefully, by now, you are starting to see that proper sleep is an integral part of your fat loss program. Let me share my top 4 tips for a great night's sleep:

1. Make sure the room is dark - and by dark, I mean pitch black.

Turn off bedside lights, alarm clocks (cover these) and make sure no street lights are shining through the gaps beside the blind. You may even want to invest in a black-out blind. Most people notice an immediate improvement in length and quality of sleep from this step alone.

2. Aim for 8 - 9.5 hours of sleep each night

While we can survive on less than this, we cannot thrive. There is no medal in life for being the person who gets the least sleep. When you sleep more, not only does your weight loss improve but so will your productivity the next day.

3. Ensure you have consistent wake and sleep times

Consistency in the aftermath and sleep times are essential for the body to get into a healthy rhythm. Inconsistent wake and sleep times throw us into a constant state of mild jet lag. We have all experienced the mild jet lag effects of traveling into a time zone only a few hours away. No one wants to feel this way in their everyday life.

4. Be sure to "unplug' the hour before bed

That means turn off the television and computer. Give the brain some time to unwind and slow down. Try reading a good book or writing in a journal.

I have seen stubborn fat begin to shift when patients start getting a good night's sleep. Getting enough sleep is the missing link that stops or slows down many people's weight loss.

So, follow the four steps above - you'll love the results.

Chapter 5: Putting It All Together

Cardio

Cardio is an integral part of your fitness. There are lots of different guidelines out there. For basic competence, it's recommended to do 30 minutes of moderate cardio five days a week or 20 minutes of vigorous or more intense cardio three times a week. You don't need to do more unless you're training for a fitness event like a race or you're trying to lose weight.

The good news? You don't need to do the 20 to 30 minutes all at once (Although, personally, I find it easier to do one workout a day as opposed to two or more).

There are two types of cardio: endurance and bursts.

Bursts are precisely what it sounds, short bursts of energy. They're also typically pretty intense as you're pushing yourself to your maximum exertion. Any sprinting or plyometrics (I'll show you plyometrics in the exercise breakdown section) are considered cardio bursts.

Over 40 Note - a plyometric can also be known as a ploy. Plyos are fast, energetic bursts of energy where you're working for short periods of time at your maximum ability. For example, stand up and raise your arms above your head. Jump up as high as you can ten times in a row. That's a plyometric move.

Endurance is more about doing cardio over an extended period. Depending on your current activity level, tolerance for you can mean anywhere from 10 minutes or more. However, persistence relates typically to doing a cardio activity such as running, biking, hiking, and swimming for 30 minutes and up. Brisk walking can also be included here.

Now, when you're working on improving your endurance or distance, you'll want to follow the long and slow theory. That's because you can't push yourself to work at your maximum heart rate for that long. Instead, you'll want to work out at 65-75% of your maximum capacity, or the fastest that you know that you can run. Otherwise, you'll burn out and won't be able to go the distance.

Think of it as pacing yourself. You don't want to sprint or go top speed when you go far; you just can't keep that kind of pace for long periods of time. Many coaches will have you base your effort on your actual heart rate. The best way to determine your exertion rate is to wear a heart rate monitor.

And if you can't afford a heart monitor or don't want to wear one, here's another option to try. When you're doing endurance training, you know you're going at the right place when you can talk. I'm not saying you can hold a full on a conversation (if you can, you're probably not working hard enough). It should take some extra effort to talk, but if you find you can't speak at all, back off the intensity until you can.

Now, when you are doing cardio bursts or plyos, you shouldn't be able to talk at all because you're working at your maximum intensity. So if you can, you're not working hard enough, and you need to ramp it up.

While this isn't a total fool-proof method, it does work pretty well at keeping you in your target heart range.

Keep this in mind when doing any cardio workout. Whenever I have you doing a burst (sprint or plyo), work to your maximum. Try to talk. It should come out in ragged, breathless bursts. When you're doing more endurance work, you should be able to speak with just a little extra effort.

Strength Training

A lot of women aren't quite as familiar with strength training as they are with cardio. And let's face it: years ago, strength training was seen as more of a man's workout than for women. Women feared to bulk up, and there wasn't anyone to show them the way.

But that's all in the past.

Strength training should be an integral part of your fitness routine. It helps build muscle mass and keeps your bones healthy.

Considering that women are at a much higher risk for osteoporosis and osteopenia, why wouldn't you do it?

Contrary to the beliefs of the past, strength training (also known as resistance training) doesn't cause us to bulk up; it keeps us looking long and lean. Not to mention it has a beautiful side benefit: when you build muscle, you burn A LOT more calories. Even while you're at rest; just sitting around watching TV.

Let me explain. Yes, it's true; a pound is a pound is a pound. A pound of fat may weigh the same as a pound of muscle, but that pound is in no way equal. That's because the tissue is much denser than fat, so it makes you look leaner. But the best part? A pound of flesh burns about 50 calories a day. Fat burns a paltry two. Yes, you read that right. Just two calories. If that doesn't give you the incentive to move it, I don't know what will. You can eat more! And still, lose the weight. Bonus!

To get more out of your strength training, here are my five tips.

Tip #1 - Avoid the machines. If you're a gym gal, stay clear of the devices and head to the free weights. Weight machines tend to work on one isolated muscle. Plus, they typically have us moving in a way we don't usually run. Instead, use the free weights.

Tip #2 - Intervals are the way to go. To get the biggest bang for your buck, interval training is critical. By interval training, I mean mixing cardio in with your strength training. Why? By mixing the two you'll keep your heart rate elevated, thereby increasing the calories you burn.

Tip #3 - You need to feel it. Don't think you can only lift 2 or 3-pound weights; the key to getting results is to make sure that you can feel the resistance. So don't be afraid to move up. That said, when you're doing intervals, you're going to use lighter weights. For my workouts, I recommend at least three-pound weights but no more than five. If you don't feel like these are enough, you're not pushing yourself during the cardio portion enough, or you're doing the reps way too fast.

Tip #4 - Slow it down. When you lift weights, I want you to concentrate on the lowering of the weight. That's right, the lowering, or "negative" as it's called, causes an eccentric contraction. Don't worry about the term, just know that particular decrease is the most crucial part of the exercise. Eccentric contraction means muscle lengthening.

I can't tell you how many times I see people lifting too fast. If you do it too quickly, you're missing out on the resistance as you lower the weight which is more than half of the exercise!!!! So you're doing yourself a disservice. The best way to make sure you're doing resistance training at a proper speed is to do it in two counts. Two counts up, two counts down. So in your head, number 1, two as you lift and then 1, two as you lower the weight or position. In other words, SLOW DOWN!!!

Tip #5 - Don't be afraid to increase. Some experts, such as Cosgrove, suggest letting the number of repetitions dictate how much weight you start with. Pick a weight that you can lift eight times, maybe 10, but probably not more than 12 consecutive times.

Physical fitness is set higher than the health fitness standards, and they require a more intense exercise program. Physically fit people of all ages have the freedom to enjoy most of life's daily and recreational activities.

Your objectives will determine the fitness program you decide to use. If the primary aim of your fitness program is to lower the risk of disease, attaining the usual fitness standards will provide substantial health benefits. If, however, you want to participate in vigorous fitness activities, achieving a high physical fitness standard is recommended. This book gives both health fitness and physical fitness standards for each fitness test so you can personalize your approach.

Chapter 6: Tips to Initiate Change

Make it enjoyable and fun

You deserve to enjoy your exercise. Even though you deserve you feel like you're thirty years old, you don't have to work out like you're thirty. You've lived a good fifty years now, and that means you can reward yourself with a little enjoyable exercise.

There is plenty of exercises out there that is enjoyable and fun. Spend some time finding an activity that you enjoy. You don't have to slave away running on a treadmill if that just sounds like torture to you. Sure that might be the fastest way to get your exercise, but who says you need to get your exercise fast if you hate every second of it.

One of the things I've learned throughout my years is that if you hate exercising, you won't feel very motivated to use every day. If you look forward to applying, you won't have to fight with yourself to get it done. Mainly it doesn't feel like a chore, it feels like an exciting and happy part of your day.

Let me give you a few examples to think about while you think about how to make your exercise enjoyable and fun. One of the things I've always really enjoyed is walking with friends. I have two close friends that I enjoy walking with after work a few times during the week. We used to work together, and our jobs have taken us different directions through the years, but we've stayed good friends by walking along in the afternoons.

Another thing that I've enjoyed doing, as I've gotten older is playing tennis. My daughter played when she was younger, and I always loved watching her play. I thought that I'd like to learn how but stayed away from the idea for a long time until finally, I decided to try an adult league at our local athletic club. It was a beginner's league with other women just like myself. We all knew the basics of the sport, but no one was a star.

It was fun, and I've enjoyed playing in the league every year for the six weeks they do the program. I don't have any hidden fantastic talent by any means, but I enjoy playing, it gets me on my feet for a few hours a couple of times a week, and I've met new people that I enjoy being with.

So get out there and find some workouts that you enjoy and will give you the chance to have a bit of fun. Exercise doesn't have to be tedious and cumbersome. If you aren't looking forward to your workout every day, do something to change it up and enjoy yourself. I promise that if you have a workout program that you experience, you will be much more motivated to stay with it in the long run.

Make it a priority

There are a couple of different aspects to making this trick work for you. It is hard to make exercise fit into your daily schedule – I know. Because it is hard to schedule your practice into your day, there are a couple of things you can do to help ensure that it happens.

First, consider carefully when you schedule your workout. Schedule your workout just like you would anything else that you find a high priority. That way nothing else and no excuse can get between you and your workout. Your workout can't be something that can be skipped or tossed to the side if something else comes up.

With that being said, I will suggest that if possible you workout in the morning. I understand that doesn't work for everyone and with every kind of exercise. Here's the reason I suggest working out in the morning. If you exercise in the morning, then there are fewer excuses you can't do it. You won't find yourself saying that you are too tired from a long day at work, or other things won't come up that pull you away. The only thing you'll be fighting is your bed and laziness, which I understand can be persuasive at times; however, as I age I find it harder and harder to sleep in any way.

The only drawback to working out in the morning is that getting together with friends is more laborious, classes aren't always offered, going to the gym before work can be challenging, etc., so if you aren't working out at home or alone, it can be somewhat of a challenge.

The most important part is that you sit down and think about how you can make your workouts a right priority in your day. You have to find the time in your day that works when you will have minimal excuses. I won't say to see a time with no excuses because that time doesn't exist. There will always be a time when you have some reason or another, but there are sometimes that are better than others.

Change your attitude about exercise

I think this is one of the biggest things that I've learned over the years, and probably one of the most critical pieces of advice I can give just about anyone. I gained perhaps ten years ago, but it's never too late for anyone that exercise isn't something to dread and isn't something to hate. In fact, the practice should be part of everything we do.

I haven't always been one of those people that looked forward to my daily exercise routine, but I am now. We already talked about finding ways to enjoy and love the kind of exercise you do, but it's more than just that. It's about finding ways to incorporate training into all the little parts of your life. Instead of looking for ways to get around practice, find ways to add activity to your life.

Let me give you some examples to help you see what I mean. I mentioned earlier that I have grandkids that are relatively young. My daughter has just started them in some of the city sports leagues like soccer. Going to their games during the seasons is hilarious.

Some of the other parents and grandparents may think I'm crazy for doing that, but I also burn quite a few calories by doing that, and indeed it's not that hard. I'm just walking on a level surface watching the game. The time moves quickly, and I don't realize the time has moved as soon as it has. My daughter has joined me in the walking after asking me what I'm doing, so I'm not alone in my exercise, and I have someone to chat with.

Another example includes using the stairs instead of escalators and elevators. I don't have that chance every day, but whenever the opportunity arises, I always take the stairs instead of the lazy alternative. Especially when staying at a hotel or going through an airport. Take advantage of any opportunity to walk a little more. If you're in a hurry, just walk a little faster, you probably will beat the elevator anyway when you consider the stops and wait times.

There are many opportunities to add exercise to your day if you stop and think about it. From walking to the mailbox and searching for the closest parking spot at the grocery store, we can be a pretty lazy society if we want to, but only changing your attitude to one that seeks the opportunity to exercise daily as much as possible is one that will help you in the long run.

Journal about it

This trick doesn't work for everyone, but it has worked wonders for me. I first started using this method as something to help me stick to my new year's resolutions, which weren't always related to weight loss and working out, but often were.

When we think about the traditional journals, we often think about something that is bound with paper inside, but it doesn't need to be that traditional. We have many different ways in society today that you could keep a journal. It could be something on your phone if that's the way that you keep track of your life.

There are some different apps you could download or maybe even already have downloaded that would be excellent for keeping track of your goals and exercise routines both for the days and weeks. When you have things written down in a place that is easy for you to refer to, you can check with yourself and make notes about how you are doing and also see back to how you have done.

I don't know if you are anything like me, but it's easy to forget from week to week how things are progressing with your workouts. I don't have the memory I used to when I was younger, and it may be that things are just blending from day to day because I do a lot of the same things. If I take the time to write words down, I can easily remember what I did and how I did.

I'm not perfect with my workouts and some days it's nice to be able to refer back and see where I can improve and what goals I need to make to continue to grow. By writing the goals down, I can often apply back to them and remind myself what I am working towards.

The traditional journal, the phone, a tablet, a small notepad, etc. are all ways you could consider keeping track of your workouts and your goals. It helps to keep you accountable for something. Whatever method you choose, make it something that you are happy with and something that you will look at often. It needs to be close to where you work out and with you when you exercise.

Join forces

I already mentioned earlier that I enjoy walking with a few of my closest friends and that even though we no longer work together, we have still stayed close as friends because we walk together. This is one of those things that as we get older, we can enjoy. I don't know about others out there, but I enjoy a good chat with friends, and there's nothing better than taking that conversation out on a walking path.

So I strongly recommend getting together with some good friends and making it a regular thing. You won't regret it. It doesn't have to be walking, but it seems to be an easy thing to do because you can always walk and talk at the same time. However, I have known other women to join together and do yoga clubs, cycling, etc. It's just beautiful to have other people to do exercise with.

We are women, and we don't like to do things by ourselves. It's true when men make fun of us for going to the bathroom together. Regardless of whether or not you are one of those kinds of women, you can still organize some type of club or group of women in your area to get together and do something. If you don't want to be the head of the group because you don't feel like you have the skill to teach, you can get everyone together and take a class at the local rec center or health club. It will probably cost a little money, but this is your health we're talking about – it's worth a small cost.

It doesn't always have to be friends either. I keep going back to walking, but I also enjoy walking with my spouse on weekend evenings in the summer when it's nice outside. He and I just walk the neighborhood after dinner during dusk. It's just an excellent way to end the day. It's almost like a date, but it's free, and we get to spend the time enjoying each other's company and catching up on each other's day.

He and I also offer to babysit our grandkids a couple of times a month so our kids and their spouses can have a date night and let me tell you babysitting our grandchildren can be a workout by itself. Now this kind of goes back to that attitude about exercise thing. I have had thoughts about just renting a movie and getting fast food for the kids. It would make a much more natural night for grandma and grandpa. However, it's much more fun for everyone when we play tag in the backyard and hide and seek.

All of these things are about getting together with others and finding ways to exercise together. It helps to have others encourage you while you support them.

Make it a competition

This is such a fun way to exercise. I don't know about you, but I am not extremely competitive, but there is a little competitive streak inside me that makes it a little fun.

I mentioned earlier that I joined a tennis league in town, which has a competition every year, and that is always fun, but I am not talking about that kind of game.

The kind of competition I am talking about involves getting a few people that are also similarly trying to workout as you. They should even be trying to make working out a part of their everyday life. Maybe they are trying to lose weight and eat healthy, too. You'll have to decide the perimeters of the competition.

Reward yourself

Before we talk about external rewards, let's take just a minute to talk about the internal compensation that doing all the exercise and working out can bring you. If you stop and take a moment to remember that you are prolonging your life and increasing the time that you will have with family and friends, it is a reward in and of itself. I love savoring those thoughts every day of my life. It is nice to remember that by taking care of my health and keeping my body younger, I am giving myself time and energy to spend with my wondering and beautiful grandchildren that I wouldn't have otherwise. I know that it is worth that every time I spend with them. I love seeing them grow older and that is a reward.

It also just feels good to exercise. Although it is hard to get out of bed, and sometimes hard to even get my shoes tied in the afternoon after a long day at work, I remind myself that after a good workout, I will feel better and be stronger. The endorphins and other hormones that are released from the exercise give me such a happy feeling that it's all worth it. I am always glad after I exercise, that I have to remind myself beforehand to push the excuses aside and get through the initial struggles.

That all being said, some external rewards are excellent sometimes, too. Through the years, I have set up rewards to keep myself motivated during those rough times. This is something that will help you to stay motivated along the way. I am not suggesting that you do substantial rewards every time you lose a pound or do one workout, but I have learned that giving yourself little rewards can give you the motivation to keep going through the hard times, so what kinds of awards are we talking about then?

Although we aren't talking about diets in this book, I would strongly recommend never giving yourself a food reward. Food rewards are just wrong in so many ways. You might try and just giving yourself a food reward once or twice, but it's so easy to do once that you'll do it over and over again and you just don't want to fall into that trap – trust me. You are undoing everything that you worked so hard to do with your workouts, and it's just not worth it.

Instead, there are so many other great things out there that you can reward yourself with instead that are worth your time and money. Spend your energy there instead of food, and you'll be glad you did. Choose your rewards early on, so you know what you are working towards. It will help to give you the motivation to understand why you are working so hard through those days when it feels so hard to get out of bed and to the gym.

Start by thinking up small rewards. These kinds of awards are for the end of the month or the end of the week. They don't need to be anything significant. Think of something you know you want, like a book that is being released soon or a new pair of shoes that you've been dying to buy. Tell yourself you can't get them until you've met an individual goal. This doesn't need to be a big goal; maybe it's just two or three weeks of straight exercising.

Once you've met your goal, reward yourself by buying the shoes or downloading the book onto your tablet and indulging by reading for a few hours. Whatever the reward is, let yourself relish in the premium for a time. Savor the moment and love yourself a little before moving on to whatever the next goal and reward are. Remind yourself that you are committed to your exercise and being a new and healthy person.

The longer and more significant goals deserve bigger and healthier rewards. You'll need to sit and think a little longer about what kind of compensation you want to get for yourself once you meet those goals. It could mean a full day at the spa being pampered and taken care of. If that's not your thing, maybe you've been eying some new clothes to go with that new healthier body. I don't know what kind of reward fits your lifestyle or your personality, but think about it and decide carefully what you deserve. Make it enticing and inviting enough that you will stay motivated enough to work hard and make it toward your goal.

Rewards are all about giving you something to look forward to when you reach the end. You know yourself better than anyone else. Thus you should be the one to set the goals and define your rewards.

Make it cost something

I briefly mentioned shelling out some money for your health a few chapters ago, and we're going to go into a little more detail here, sometimes if you make your workouts cost something, you feel a bit more motivation to get them done. Let's talk about why that happens and a few examples of how you can do that.

First of all, if you pay in advance for anything in life, you are far more likely to attend because you don't want to waste the money. It's that simple. It works the same with your workouts, so if you pay cash for a gym membership, a class, etc. you are more likely to attend because you will feel guilty about wasting the money otherwise. You don't want to see the money go down the drain so you will do something about it.

Let me say something about gym memberships. I have had a little trouble with gym memberships in the past. I signed up for a gym membership that had a year contract. I thought it would be convenient to have them just pull the membership fee from my bank out each month. I never even saw the monthly fee. I went faithfully for the first few months, but then I stopped going. I can't also really remember the reason why, but I am sure there was a slew of good excuses.

Because I wasn't responsible for the monthly payments and it just automatically came out of my checking account, I didn't feel that guilt. Forgetting about it was easy. I have even known some people who pay off their gym memberships for the whole year all at once, so my suggestion to you is that you keep it your responsibility to take cash or a check into the gym every month.

It will keep you accountable and make you feel guilty if you aren't using the membership.

There are lots of options out there for you to look into for classes and exercise programs. If you aren't one for a gym, don't. I don't belong to a gym anymore and with good reason. I didn't use the gym as I should have, but I learned that the gym wasn't my kind of place to workout. It works for a lot of people, and that's great. If the gym is for you, then, by all means, use their facilities.

The local rec centers offer lots of classes that are reasonably priced and give you lots of opportunities to try new things and meet new people. You can also check with athletic clubs, too see what they are offering. That's where I found the tennis league.

Ultimately, you have to remember that a little cost and money is nothing compared to your health. You have to be willing to make a few sacrifices here and there with your recreational activities or other things to ensure that you are healthy and that your body is where you want.

Give yourself a "lazy" day

The title of this trick perhaps is a little misleading. I don't want you to think of this day as your cheat day or the day you don't have to do anything. However, we all need a day during the week when we don't have to work as hard. Most of us consider that the weekend, right? Sometimes we get two days during the week when we are a little lazier.

I know that for me I usually consider Sunday my lazy day during the week. I go to work and work pretty hard during the week Monday through Friday. Then Saturday is a pretty rough day for me, too. I usually spend my Saturday outside working in the garden or mowing the grass or even the flowerbeds, too. I can't think of a Saturday that isn't spent doing something productive. I clean the house, also, so also if I'm not outside, I'm doing things inside as well. Then it seems like my Sunday is a lot more laid back than the other days. I try to give myself a day to catch up on the other things around the house. It's not that Sunday is entirely unproductive, but it does feel a little more laid back than the other days.

When it comes to my exercise and workouts, I kind of plan my schedule the same way. I plan more rigorous workouts Monday through Friday. Even though the days are busier, I am also already up and moving those days. It is easy to add another thing to the day because I am already up and out the door. I walk with my two good friends every day after work for somewhere between forty-five minutes and an hour. We meet in between work and dinner with our spouses, so it works out well.

I also add a small workout in the later evening after dinner but before bed. It's during that time when most people are watching television. I have my favorite television shows, too, but I have added an element of exercise into my evening while I watch them. During the opening theme songs and commercials, I do different tasks just to add a little something extra.

Every morning when I first wake-up I also do a small thirty workout, too. It's short and varies from day to day depending on what I have time for, but it gives me something to start my day. I have always felt that starting my day with exercise gives me extra energy and gets my body moving and awake. I enjoy the feelings I get when I start my day with use, so even if I can only get twenty minutes of rigorous training, I will still run down to our basement and use.

Saturdays are one of my favorite days because I get a really good workout. I always give myself an hour or so to work out hard. Again this exercise varies, but I run on a treadmill, ride a stationary bike, lift small weights, circuit train, do workout videos, etc.

Okay, now let's talk about my lazy day since that's what this chapter is really about. Sunday is my lazy day, but that doesn't mean I don't do anything. I still try and do something, just something small. Sunday I usually always stretch extensively and then do a little yoga and breathing exercises. I took a yoga class, and I am acutely aware that yoga can be an extensive workout if you want it to be. However, the yoga that I do is more like desperate stretching – maybe I should call it that.

I also try to use my pedometer on Sundays and ensure that I walk at least 10K steps on Sundays, which equates to somewhere in the neighborhood of around four miles. I know that might sound like a lot, but you'd be surprised at how many steps you walk just by walking around your house throughout the day. By strapping on the pedometer you'll probably have to walk more to get to 10K, but not too many more. You'll have to start pushing yourself when you want to walk more than 10K.

My real point with all of this is that we all deserve a day when we relax. No one should be required to workout seven days a week. You will burn yourself out quickly if you don't cut yourself a little break and give yourself a lazy day at least once a week. However, that lazy day doesn't mean you get to sit on the couch all day and eat potato chips and French fries counteracting everything you did all week.

Instead consider giving yourself a lazy day that still is somewhat productive, but feels good. You'll keep your motivation high while even giving yourself the results you are looking for.

Bring your media

Have you ever been to the gym and been stuck watching a soap opera because you just happened to be there at the time of day when every single channel was showing soaps? Oh wait, there was one other channel that was showing something different than a soap opera and then was a sports channel, but it was the middle of the morning, and the only thing that was on was some poker tournament that no one cared about.

I mean the least the gym could do was find the news network, right? I mean there are stations out there that play the news all day long aren't there? I think that's one of the reasons I don't have a gym membership anymore. I couldn't stand going to the gym because I couldn't ever get used to what was on the televisions. I don't know if that's changed over the years, but I still probably wouldn't go.

Even if you aren't going to the gym, it's worth investing and finding ways to bring your media to your workouts. Here is why. You'll enjoy your workout so much more if you can watch, read or listen to what you want. Here are some ways and things you can do to make that happen.

First thing is the most accessible – music. Music is a beautiful way to get yourself in the mood and to stay in the atmosphere during your workout. You can find great music that will get you pumped up to exercise. There are great playlists that already exist if this is new and you are struggling to find music. You can also connect with individual artists that are known to be good for workout music. It's easy to put in some headphones any mp3 player and get to work. You can also blast the music over some speakers if you are in the comfort of your own home.

The other suggestion I have with music is to change it often. Don't keep the same playlist for weeks on end. Change it up. As simple as this sounds, it will help to keep you motivated to listen to your new music. You will know that you have a new playlist and you'll be excited to hear the original music the next time you have a workout. It seems simple and something so easy, but trust me it does work, so change your music often and keep things circulating through to keep things fresh.

If you are doing something somewhat stationary like a treadmill or a stationary bike you can consider watching a television show, movie or reading a tablet. I have recently really enjoyed reading my tablet while riding my stationary bike. I try not to do anything tough, just a nice steady ride while I read. It's a good workout, while also reading a good book. I can usually ride for twice as long if I'm reading. If I'm running on my treadmill, I can watch television. I enjoy do that, too. It makes the time go by much faster. I don't realize that thirty minutes have gone by.

Because I own my tablet and have these things at my house, I can choose what I want to watch and what I want to read while I run and ride. It makes my ride and runs much more enjoyable to me. Then I'm not watching a terrible soap opera – no offense to anyone who enjoys soap operas –or watching as every second passes on the treadmill just waiting for thirty minutes to cross so I can feel like I've done my workout for the day.

It's nice to pick and have your media because then you can feel like you have control over your private workout. You don't have to own your treadmill or stationary bike to make the exercise enjoyable. If you are going to the gym, you can still enjoy your workout and control the media.

Use your phone, tablet,etc. to control the media if you aren't

enjoying what's broadcast in front of you. Create playlists before you go so that you can enjoy every second and minute of your workout. Change those playlists often to keep things new and fresh to keep you motivated through every minute of your exercise.

Don't judge yourself based on the scale

This is a tough thing to do, but you can't always look at the number on the scale and decide yourself. It's so easy to get caught up on what is flashing before you each time you step on the scale, but you have to try very hard not to let it overwhelm you.

If you have to, get rid of your scale altogether. For a long time, I didn't own a level for that reason. My husband was the one who had the idea to get rid of the size, and as hard as it was to live without one, I can admit now that he was right. There are a few reasons that judging yourself based on the scale is detrimental.

The first is that fat and muscle weigh differently. Muscle weighs more than fat does. If you burn fat but gain muscle you will gain weight, so depending on the types of workouts you are doing, you might be building more muscle, but burning fat at the same time, which would cause you to feel and look great. However, you'd gain weight if you stepped on the scale. If I were in that situation, which I have been in, I would be devastated by the numbers on the scale.

When I was in that situation, I felt awful, because I had been working so hard. I'd be dieting, exercising and depriving myself of so many things that I loved. I expected to see significant changes on the scale, so to see the opposite of what I thought was devastating. Instead of looking at myself in the mirror and seeing the results I wanted in the body staring back at me, I could only look at the numbers on the scale.

That was when my husband suggested we ditch the scale.

Another reason to steer clear of your scale is that your weight fluctuates so frequently. I have learned that from one day to the next my weight can change two pounds or more. I don't really know the science behind that, but I have seen it on so many occasions. Experts will tell you that it's better just to weigh yourself every couple weeks or even less like once a month. That will give you a better indication of where your weight stands.

There are so many tricks and things people tell you about when and how to weigh yourself. It's worst to consider yourself at night, best in the morning. Weigh yourself before you've eaten anything; get an expensive scale to get an accurate reading, etc. All of that doesn't matter.

The numbers flashing up at you on the scale don't matter. Look at yourself in the mirror. That's what matters. The way that you fit in your clothes. That's what matters. The way you feel about yourself. That's what matters.

Don't be afraid to try new things

My final trick and suggestion to keeping motivated are to try new things.

Don't be scared to give a few new things a try now and then. I know we are a little bit older – notice I didn't say old. It's easy to get stuck in our ways and feel comfortable with the things we've done our whole lives, but it's also not as enjoyable.

We've already talked about making your workouts enjoyable so that we won't hash that again, but I will strongly recommend finding some new things in your area to try that you may never have thought about before.

You can find new things almost anywhere you go. Your local rec center will have classes and leagues in many different sports and activities that you can join, some will only be offered at certain times of the years, but there is bound to be something provided at any given time of the year that you can join and try. The great thing about the classes they offer is that there will always be a beginner level of the course, so you won't ever have to feel that you are stuck with people who know the sport or activity at a different level than you.

I was always able to take classes or join activities with people who were at the same level as me – novices. The teachers still took things very slow and never expected anything from any of us. They knew that we were there for the first time, with little to no knowledge of the sport or activity. Let me share with you an example of a class I took.

There might be a yoga class offered at the local community college that you can sign-up for. Our community college here in town offers many different courses to the community on nights and weekends that I've considered. My daughter convinced me to take a couple with her a few years ago. Here's that joining together thing again. Neither of us would have made the classes alone, but together we tried Pilates, and it wasn't too bad. I don't think either of us fell in love, but we both had a good time and enjoyed the workout twice a week in the evenings.

Several of the things we talked in this book applied to taking that class. We paid money for it, so we felt committed. It was something new that neither of us had tried before, and we had each other to help feel motivated. We've talked about doing something like that again in a future semester.

The most important thing is not to be afraid when you are asked or confronted with new ideas. Try them and give them a shot. You might find something new that you love. You might not. You also might find a hidden talent that you never knew you had. Regardless of what you see, you even might make some new friends or rekindle and enrich relationships with old friends.

Stick with it

Exercising and working out doesn't have to be the bane of your existence. You don't have to feel like you hate every minute you remember you have to workout. Instead, there are many different things you can do to enjoy yourself and motivate yourself to keep with it and stay strong through your workouts.

One of the most important things I've done both through the years and continue to do now is changing my attitude about exercise and working out in general. I no longer feel that task is that part of the day when I roll my eyes and sigh with relief when it's over. Instead, I look forward to it and get excited about it. I feel motivated about every minute both before and after.

Educate yourself regarding the benefits of a healthy lifestyle and subscribe to several important health, fitness, and wellness subscription or books. The more you read, understand, and then start living a wellness lifestyle, the more your core values will change. At the time you should, you should also break relationships with individuals who are unwilling to change with you.

Procrastination – People seem to think that tomorrow, next week, or after the holiday is the best time to start change.

Tips to Initiate Change – Ask yourself: Why wait until tomorrow when you can start changing today? Lack of motivation is a critical factor in procrastination.

Preconditioned cultural beliefs. If we accept the idea that we are a product of our environment, our cultural views and our physical surroundings pose significant barriers to change.

In Salzburg, Austria people of both genders and all ages use bicycles as a primary mode of transportation. In the United States, few people other than children ride bikes.

Chapter 7: Getting Your Mind in the Game

Before you embark upon any life-changing goal, what do most people do?

They make a plan. They prepare themselves mentally. Without this sort of mental preparation, the mind doesn't have the motivation to take on the task. You could pick any diet plan, any exercise routine, but if you aren't on board mentally, none of it will work.

This is the most important chapter of this book. If you take nothing else from this book, I urge you to pay close attention to this: *Your mind has everything to do with why you are currently overweight.* It is not your genetics; it is not the condition of wheat products today, it is not because you are addicted to food. While all of those things may play a part, the reason you are overweight is that of what's going on with you mentally and emotionally.

Think of the battle that goes on every day -- the need to be healthy versus the need to fill the void in your being with food. Just thinking about losing weight might bring about a feeling of resistance or dread.

Your weight will be a constant battle that you will never win if you don't comfort that hurting thing inside you that makes you eat.

There are so, so many reasons people gain weight. Perhaps you were molested at an early age, and you have surrounded your body in fat as a means of protection or to shield you from harmful attention. Maybe you don't think you deserve to be fit and healthy and are stuck in a cycle of self-loathing because your father wasn't in the picture and you don't believe you are worthy of love. Maybe you are comforting yourself with food for a variety of reasons and therefore consider yourself 'addicted' to food. Whatever it may be, you must give it a name, and hug that crying child inside. Until that fear or hurt is brought to light, given a name and soothed, it will continue to scream for attention.

When we have been injured emotionally in the past and turn to food for comfort, we tend to justify it. Those justifications are what is keeping us in the body fat prison, and it has to stop. We are often too easy on ourselves, which in the end will only destroy us. Justifying our weight with excuses -- too busy, too tired, too whatever. In life, as in weight loss, we just experience CHANGE when we are willing to step out of our comfort zone.

Leaving our comfort zone doesn't mean making HUGE changes like crazy exercise routines and strict diets that leave us hungry and angry. It just requires making one small difference a day in the direction of good health. Baby steps! Because humans tend to move in the direction of what feels right, just PICK FOODS AND PHYSICAL ACTIVITIES THAT YOU ENJOY. Those small achievements each day feeling right, and you will want to continue to explore good.

But there is another mental/emotional roadblock that must be overcome -- and that is the overall impression you might have towards weight loss. I want you to think about weight loss for a moment. Did you get a sinking feeling in your chest or a negative feeling of any kind? If so, then your mind is not YET in the game. Your account is in resistance for any number of reasons, and when you resist the idea of the hard work that might accompany weight loss, then ANYTHING YOU DO to get there will fail eventually. Law of Attraction is not just for romance novels -- it is the force in place across the universe that makes things happen. You can use it in to manifest what you want in your life, which I will discuss in depth in the following chapter. The theory of 'alignment' refers to whether the life you are living NOW is lined up, so to speak, with the best life you can be living (often referred to as 'The Higher Self'). Once we can change the way we think about losing weight, we will then be able to attract what we want and therefore line up with our intended best self -- a happy, healthy, fit person!

The fight against fat does not have to be something we struggle with -- think of it more as chasing after happiness. When you feel that desperation to lose weight, it causes resistance in your body. Because there is such a tight relationship between mind and body, the body will then resist the change that you apparently feel so strongly about!

The best thing you can for yourself right now is to meditate (see chapter Visualization and Meditation) and make a plan. Weight loss will be achievable the moment you believe it is! Never listen to your best friend or your sister's method to lose weight. It won't work for you because you are your person with your personal issues. Focus on what YOU think will work for you, and it will.

Sometimes, affirmations help me get my mind in the game. Feel free to use my statements below or write your own. Repeat these to yourself every morning. Every. Single. Morning.

1. Your inner child is safe now. You are a grownup and are in charge now. No one can hurt you anymore.

2. I love myself, even if no one else does. And I am the only one who can make this change.

3. I am strong, and I am worthy of love.

4. Getting my body back into its initially intended state is something I do for me because I love myself.

5. Getting my body back into its proposed state initially will bring me joy.

6. Every reasonable step I take brings me one step closer to pleasure.

7. My inner child needs hugs, not food. I will hug that scared, sad child inside and give it the love it needs.

8. Anyone can be fat. Being fat is easy. Getting control of my mind and body is a great accomplishment.

9. Greatness involves risk. I am ready to take the chance.

10. Even if I never lose another pound, I love myself and don't blame myself for this extra weight.

Once you can break the cycle, you will love yourself and lose weight for yourself. It will come easy. You will no longer need 'comfort foods' or want to celebrate with food. Food will become what it is intended to be -- nourishment and nothing else.

Trying to lose weight without getting your head in the game will never, ever work. You need to visualize, meditate, and heal whatever injury inside that is making you overeat.

The Law of Attraction and Alignment

To manifest your goals in life, it might benefit you to turn to your spiritual side to achieve the best results.

Each of us is born 'perfect.' For the most part, when we are very young, nothing has happened to us that might affect us emotionally, or at least that we are aware of yet. Each day, we move slowly toward our 'higher selves,' which is your correct, best, most pure self. The self that we were born to be.

At some point, we might experience some emotional pain, which causes us to begin to deviate from the higher self. Perhaps we lost a family member, or our parents suffered a divorce. Maybe we were mistreated in some way which caused psychological damage. Maybe we were even born with an illness that confuses our reality. It's also familiar to learn misguided patterns of unhealthy behavior from our very own parents and grandparents. As a result, we might begin making bad choices like using drugs or alcohol, making the wrong kinds of friends, hurting our relationships, and even abusing food -- all behavior that will take us further and further away from the best person we were meant to be.

If our higher self is our true calling, then happiness will occur when we become that self. Each step we take toward that elusive person will, therefore, in theory, feel good. Our bodies are beautiful things that tell us whenever we are doing something that isn't good for us -- GUILT is an excellent example of this. When we do something like eating food that isn't good for us, our bodies let us know through guilt that we aren't making the best choice. When we overeat, we feel uncomfortably full. And on the flip-side, when we finish a workout, our bodies are flooded with a hormone that makes us feel joyful. When we fill up on fruits and vegetables, we feel light and energetic. I'll discuss this concept further in the next chapter: "Listening to Your Body's Signals," but for now, I want you to understand how we can guide our NOW selves onto the path to the higher person.

Chasing this higher self-requires bravery. It will mean that you can't just sit back and eat whatever you want, or sit on the couch and expect to reach that particular place. You will have to remove yourself from your comfort zone. That, in and of itself, will feel good. Deciding to will feel good. Each time you make a positive movement toward your higher self, your body will let you know. You will feel right about it!

Allow me, if you will, to offer a spiritual analogy that might help you understand yourself better. So, you've been gaining weight steadily over the years, and your diets work for a brief time then stop. You feel bad about yourself. You dwell on everything you're doing WRONG that makes you gain weightght. Imagine, now, that you had an emotional bank account. You want to lose weight; you plan to cut your calories or workout more. But every time you 'mess up,' you are making a withdrawal from that emotional bank account. This happens over and over again, each time you diet. After a few years and a few dozen attempts at diets, you go bankrupt, because you've overdrawn your emotional bank account!

Instead, what you SHOULD be doing is not focusing on the withdrawals. Focus on the DEPOSITS. Every time you eat a healthy meal, you are depositing into your account. If you make enough 'deposits,' then the withdrawals don't matter. Making those emotional deposits will get your head in the game. These little deposits are gifts to yourself; small acts of self-love. Focus only on the deposits, and soon, there will be fewer withdrawals because your overall vibration will be raised and soon, your bank account will be full!

Why Deprivation Will Never Work

At some point in our history, if a person wanted to lose weight, they were encouraged to eat less and exercise more. I still hear this ancient theory today. And I am here to tell you that it is all baloney.

When your body feels deprived of nourishment, it's going to respond with cravings and some pretty intense physical symptoms. Your body is stopping you from starving. And sooner or later, you will succumb, and when you do --, you will overindulge. It's not a matter of willpower, and it doesn't make you weak. It's just human nature.

Have you ever started out the day active by having a smoothie for breakfast at 7:30 a.m., and by 10:30 a.m. you are ready to break into the office vending machine? We try, then fail, then feel bad for failing, and it's a vicious circle.

Because deprivation doesn't work. And, more importantly, it's why OTHER diets haven't worked for you. Other foods are written for other people! Only you know what kind of meals will feel like deprivation. Your dietary needs are different from others'. You need to design your plan on your own, personal needs. If the diet plan you've been following tells you-you can only eat 1200 calories a day, you are going to feel deprived. I don't care who you are. If your diet plan says you can't eat carbs (and you've always eaten carbs), you are going to feel deprived. And so on.

It's a coping strategy designed to keep us alive. And we've been fighting against this survival mechanism for decades. It's time to embrace our truths and stop setting ourselves up for imminent failure. Once you've reached your goal weight, there's one policy you need to adopt regarding food that will prevent the madness: Eat what you want, when you want, and stay when you are full.

Personally, when I think of eating less and exercising more, my body goes into panic mode. The resistance I feel too that notion feels like a tightness in my chest. It feels unpleasant even to consider. The old-fashioned methods for weight loss were misguided and torturous. They might have worked for some people for a short amount of time, but it's not a long-term solution.

We are just now beginning to understand more about food combinations and proper nutrition needed for healthy, lifelong weight maintenance, and none of it involves depriving yourself of the very food that your body needs to get through the day!

For instance, maybe you can't go entirely off carbs. Perhaps you need a slice of bread with your breakfast to feel full enough to get you through your morning. Maybe a salad will never be enough for lunch. Maybe adding protein to your mixture, and adding a side of almonds will satisfy you better. It's better to add a little something to your meal to keep you satisfied than to skip it and feel starved in a few hours. It is THEN that you will cheat because your hunger signals will be stronger than your willpower. Your body knows how to keep itself alive!

For more information about how to design your meals for optimal performance, see my chapter on Food Combinations.

Chapter 8: Metabolism Over 40

Our metabolisms have been slowing down -- way down. Personally? My decline started in my mid-twenties. I couldn't eat what I wanted anymore, and my energy was waning. My hair was starting to fall out, and my skin was thinning. Libido = nonexistent. It was terrifying. However, my normal diet routine still worked back then. I would just cut my calories to 1200 a day and workout on my stair-climber for 30 minutes a day. So, at least there was that on which I could depend.

But then I started getting older. I had my children at age 36 and 39. My body went crazy! If I had any metabolism, it was GONE by the time I hit 40. What's worse is that my old weight loss routine wasn't working anymore, and now I had baby weight that wouldn't budge. Not to mention, I became a stay-at-home mom, which limited my physical activity in a big way. I was more tired than I had ever been in my whole life.

First, I panicked. After baby #1, I was 20 lbs overweight, and then after baby #2, I was 40 pounds overweight. No matter what I tried to do, I could not lose it. The more I thought about it, the worse it got because I started stress eating. People around me in the same predicament would tell me that this was just the way it was, and there's nothing that could be done about it. A slippery slope, for sure. One I didn't want to ride down.

Does that mean we throw in the towel? Of course not. But once we learn how to adjust our typical weight loss routine to one that will work with our new hormone and metabolism changes, the scale will finally begin to move!

So I did research. Hours upon hours of research. What I learned was that there were ways to boost my metabolism, and ways to work around it to lose weight. And I got brutally honest with myself.

The bottom line about metabolism, for me, was that I was overeating. Because my metabolism had slowed so significantly, it was unable to burn off all of the extra calories I was consuming. I had to get real with myself about my nibbling.

I will eat three full meals a day, but I used to nibble in between. A handful of nuts here, a few chips there. While cooking dinner, I would nibble on the feast itself and don't even hungry by the time it was ready, yet I sat down and ate it anyway. I was utterly ignoring hunger signals. I put so much work into making it; it's not like I wasn't going to eat it! Ever done this?? Or I would double up my servings on something 'healthy,' mistakenly believing it couldn't hurt.

So, what do I do?

The first thing I discovered about how to boost my metabolism was that muscle revs it up! Each pound of muscle in your body uses six calories a day, whereas a pound of fat only uses 2. Weight training will keep your metabolism burning well after you've finished your session. So I knew the muscle-building had to become part of my plan.

I also learned that HIIT (High-Intensity Interval Training) was vital for boosting metabolic rate. Mixing up your routine will also keep your body guessing.

Thirdly, I read that water intake has a lot to do with your metabolism. I didn't know this, and I am a weak drinker, admittedly. The body needs water to burn calories. If you are even mildly dehydrated, your metabolism slows way down. So WATER would become my new best friend.

My fourth metabolism boosting change would come in the form of smaller meals. Instead of the three main meals and nibbling, I would have to switch up to having a little snack or smaller meal every three to four hours to keep things cranking.

There are also little tips for boosting metabolism with simple additions to your diet, like the addition of individual spices to your foods, like cayenne pepper, coffee or tea, 25g of fiber per day, vitamin D rich foods, iron-rich foods, and protein to every snack or meal.

So when you get around to planning your diet, a way to incorporate all of these tips might look something like this:

A sample metabolism-boosting day

7 AM Scrambled egg with spinach and a splash of hot sauce for breakfast.

10 AM Hot Green tea or coffee with a small palmful of almonds.

12 PM A salad at lunch gives you a healthy dose of fiber. Add some chopped chicken for protein.

2 PM Drink a big glass of water. You need at least 6 cups a day.

4 PM Organic grapes with a cheese stick make a great post-workout treat.

7 PM Lobster or chicken sprinkled with cayenne for dinner with a side of steamed green vegetables.

10 PM A cup of decaf green tea will soothe you before bedtime.

You might have been one of those women who, in their twenties, had no problem losing five or ten pounds. Maybe you never had to lose weight at all. Perhaps you ate whatever you wanted and worked out to tone up, instead of sweating away the pounds.

Well, this was me, for the most part.

Excuse the hair because – after all – it was 1989. I wasn't skinny by any means, but I was at a healthy weight, regardless of the fact that I ate pizza and extra value meals and pasta and bread and rarely exercised. I wore a size six or eight and continuously complained about not being a two or four. My hormones were working WITH me, back then. If I had been overindulging, I knew that cutting back the calories and working out a couple of times a week would snap me back into shape.

Those days are over. Sadly.

What worked to help us achieve a healthy weight in our twenties is irrelevant now. These are our new bodies, with new requirements, and if we want to accomplish our goals, we need to adapt and change our way of thinking.

For over-40 women, once our estrogen starts to decrease, we become prone to hormonal weight gain. Sugar causes our bodies to have an unhealthy insulin reaction. Without getting too scientific, estrogen keeps your insulin levels low. When insulin and glucose levels are also high in your blood, you are more prone to middleweight gain and Type 2 Diabetes. Also, at our age, our progesterone levels are even lower. When progesterone is high, your cortisol is lower. When the progesterone goes away during the peri-menopausal period, your cortisol raises, which also causes belly fat.

Going back to the subject of our metabolisms--we have been programmed to believe that cutting calories is the only answer to a healthy weight, when in fact, we may have only been shooting ourselves in the foot. There is research that proves that calorie-restrictive diets send your body into starvation mode. This was a protective feature of the system that saved us during the famine. Our bodies were intended to hold onto extra weight in the event of a famine, to save our lives. But the problem is, you cut calories, your body holds onto the weight, and you fail. So what happens when you fail? You give up and go back to eating without thought.

So, with all of this information under my belt, I was armed and ready to start planning what foods would help me achieve my goal. I wasn't going to restrict calories, but I would probably now be more careful of my carb intake so that I could once-and-for-all address the hormonal reasons for my middle-weight gain.

Breaking the Food Addiction

Sometimes, I am in the presence of people who STILL don't know what is right or wrong to eat. Or, they choose to ignore all of the information out there about proper nutrition. They talk about how much they want to lose weight while sitting in front of a plate of fries or while drinking soda. They'll agonize over their children's expanding middles, yet their kids' plates never see a vegetable or fruit. And who can blame them? What should we believe? A lot of the information is conflicting.

Our worlds are also a lot more complicated than in the past. It's so much easier just to ignore all the nutritional information vying for our attention and just grab something quick and easy off the supermarket shelf that you can pop in the microwave and be done with.

I am not judging, here. I am guilty of the same exact behavior. I KNOW what I need to do, but for some reason, when it comes down to it, I have a lot of trouble making a good food choice for myself. The lure of certain foods like bread, fatty meats and cheeses, pasta, salty potato chips and French fries is undeniable. After eating these 'comfort foods,' our dopamine levels are boosted, but the thrill is only temporary. (Some healthy foods boost dopamine levels like chicken, eggs, and other proteins that contain amino acids. Also seafood, apples, avocados, bananas, beets, and watermelon. I digress.)

Today's food is highly addictive. And FULL of sugar or foods that behave like sugar (CARBS) once they're in the bloodstream. Sugar stimulates the same areas of the brain as heroin and cocaine. We are addicted to it. Take it away, and you will withdraw. You might feel fatigued and foggy, irritable and lethargic. Like a drug addiction, the only way to soothe those withdrawal symptoms is to eat MORE junk. And the cycle continues.

Now, when I say 'junk food,' you might think 'fast food'as you get through a drive-thru. But there is junk food in your pantry and refrigerator, masquerading as real food. Food that my peri-menopausal body treats like candy. My significant problems were breakfast cereal, bread, raisins, diet soda, pizza, cookies, bagels. I had a lot of questions. Plus, I went out to eat about once a week. Sometimes, twice. And when I did, I had very little control over myself. It was hard to me to make a good menu choice when so many delicious options were in front of me. (See section 8: Special Occasions and Eating Out.) Every sandwich came with fries, and omelets didn't seem as fun without home fries or toast. Dining out was about to lose a lot of its appeal for me.

Junk food used to be just at the fast food restaurant or the cookie aisle in the grocery store. Now, our food is so over-processed, junk food is everywhere. Things that might have once been a healthy option should be off-limits, far ---- bread, cereals, yogurt, granola bars, bran muffins, restaurant salads, instant packets of flavored oatmeal, and the onslaught of new, 'virtuous' items that claim to be whole-grain, or trans-fat free, organic, free-range. You get the idea. Many foods that were safe in the past were now loaded with MSG or high fructose corn syrup and other additives that fuel our addiction to them. There's almost no grocery shelf food you can trust anymore.

Here's the biggest problem with battling our food addictions: unlike other habits (cigarettes, drugs, and alcohol), you cannot cut off food altogether, for obvious reasons. You can't just stop eating food. We need it to survive. And if you're a mom, maybe your kids want the bad stuff and will eat nothing resembling a whole food, so you're forced to serve food all day long that you can't eat.

So if we are eating the wrong foods for decades at a time, or the wrong portion sizes ---we will cause our bodies the same kind of damage as other addictions --- heart disease, cancer, arterial damage, *etc.* The question is --- how do we beat these unhealthy cravings when we must still indulge every day? How do we keep on track when our families want the junk? Precisely, I knew that now, as a 40-some-year-old woman, I would have to cut carbs out. And that's almost all my kids eat!

How would I ever learn to cut carbs when I crave it so much and am surround

*Vitamins, Herbs, & Supplements Oh My!*Should you be taking a vitamin? Maybe. What about supplements? Perhaps. How about herbs? Depends.Like how I answer?Probably not, but that's how I feel.To be honest, I don't have a problem with vitamins or supplements. I think they're a great way to get vital nutrients that you may not necessarily be getting from your diet.You can find lots of debate on this topic on the Internet or even discussing it with doctors and scientists. Although most agree that they are beneficial, mainly if you don't eat a healthy balanced diet. Since most people don't, or at least not every day, it's a simple and easy habit to get into to make sure that you're getting all the nutrients that your body needs. That said, in speaking with my doctor, you should buy the best quality vitamin that you can; this isn't the time to always shop by price. I like Every Woman's One Daily by New Chapter. It's filled with lots of good stuff that you won't find in your typical vitamin, plus it's formulated for women over 40. They're also probiotic and made from organic fruits, vegetables, and herbs.

Just be aware that there is truth to the statement that there can be too much of a good thing. Taking too much of any vitamin can be harmful. Just stay close to your recommend doses. So if you're making a multivitamin or supplement, you don't need to eat cereal or drink juice that contains extra calcium or folic acid.

Getting annual physical, including blood tests, pap smears, and so on fostering spiritual, social, and emotional wellness.

Tip to initiate change: Take it one step at a time.

Work on only one or two behaviors at a time so the task won't seem insurmountable.

Indifference and helplessness. A defeatist thought process often takes over, and we may believe that the way we live won't affect our health, that we have no control over our health or that our destiny is all in our genes.

Tips to imitate change: As much as 84 percent of the leading causes of death in the United States are preventable.

Rationalization. Even though people are not practicing healthy behaviors, they often tell themselves that they do get sufficient exercise, that their diet is excellent, that they have good, stable relationships, or that they don't smoke/drink/get high enough to affect their health.

Tip to initiate change: Learn to recognize when you're glossing over or minimizing a problem. You'll need to face the fact that you have a problem before you can commit to change. Your health and your life are at stake. Monitoring lifestyle habits through daily logs and then analyzing the results can help you improve self-defeating behaviors.

Illusions of invincibility.

Fat Loss vs. Weight Loss

For many years, fat loss and weight loss were used interchangeably, when in fact they are two completely separate entities.

Weight loss can be the result of the fat loss, but it can also be the result of water reduction in the body. Or, you could be losing muscle, which is not the goal. The traditional diets which required us to eat less/move more are an excellent example of this. When you starve your body of the calories it needs, you lose muscle and fat.

The ultimate goal is to lose fat while preserving as much muscle as possible. How do we do that? First of all, you have to keep your body from going into starvation mode. You need to be eating enough calories to support your activity level. I calculated that with my activity level while on Trifeca40, I would need about 100 times my body weight to accommodate my HIIT and weight training.

That way, I would not experience the hunger, cravings, and energy drain that would inevitably cause me to go back to my old ways, and probably gain twice as much weight as I wanted to lose. Why? Because I wasn't addressing the hormonal balance problem. I was merely starving myself by cutting calories.

This kind of dieting is a setup for failure. These dieters continually struggle with themselves, blaming poor willpower and self-control. There are very few people who can keep up this type of diet long-term. More than half of low-calorie dieters gain twice the weight back in the following year. I won't even go into the self-hatred and low self-esteem that eventually follows.

To meet our goal of losing fat while preserving muscle, we need to stop weighing ourselves. Get rid of your bathroom scale altogether!

Okay, maybe just hide it away in a closet. Because it is not an explicit representation of our bodies. Find a new way to calibrate your success, like measuring tape or body fat calipers. Personally, I go by clothing sizes. Once I can feel comfortable in size 8 or 10, I know I'm where I want to be.

Scales are an old-fashioned device that we have tortured ourselves with for far too long!

Gratification – People prefer instant gratification to long-term benefits.

Therefore, they will overeat (instant pleasure) instead of using self-restraint to eat moderately to prevent weight gain (long-term satisfaction).

Those who like tanning (instant gratification) avoid paying much attention to skin cancer (long-term consequence).

Tip to initiate change – Think ahead and ask yourself: How did I feel the last time I engaged in this behavior? How did it affect me? Did I feel good about the results? In retrospect, was it worth it?

Risk complacency. Consequences of unhealthy behaviors often don't manifest themselves, "If I get heart disease, I'll deal with it then. For now, let me eat, drink, and be merry."

Tip to initiate change. Ask yourself: How long do I want to live? How do I want to live? How do I want to live the rest of my life and what type of health do I want to have? What do I want to be able to do when I am 60, 70 or 80 years old?

Complexity. People think the world is too complicated, with too much to think about. If you are living the typical lifestyle, you may feel overwhelmed by everything that seems to be required to lead a healthy lifestyle, for example:

Getting Exercise

Decreasing intake of saturated and trans fats

Eating high-fiber meals and cutting total calories

Controlling using of substances

Managing stress

Wearing seat belts

Practicing safe sex

Chapter 9: The Components of the Plan

Personal Evaluation

I believe the best foundation for customizing your diet plan is to know yourself, what works for you and what doesn't, and to get it on paper. There is something about putting it in writing that makes it more official. Once you have all the information in front of you, it's easier to make right decisions about your plan.

Here's how I started: I sat down and listed everything I know about me. All of my physical limitations, emotional roadblocks, family history. It looked something like this:

I am 43 years old.

I weigh 171 lbs, and I'm 5'4".

I have a shellfish allergy and am sensitive to gluten.

I have a family history of heart disease and diabetes.

I have had two c-sections.

I am apple-shaped. Big-chested with a round tummy with thin arms and legs.

My blood type is O positive.

I am a non-smoker and drink less than three alcoholic beverages a month.

I crave sugar and fried foods.

I am fairly sedentary.

I drink no more than one bottle of water a day.

I have tendonitis in my wrists and knees.

I have gallbladder symptoms.

I believe myself to be insulin-resistant.

I cannot follow specific daily menus.

I get shaky if I don't eat every few hours.

I have WPW (heart condition) and get palpitations when my heart rate accelerates, as it would with high-impact cardio.

If I'm upset or have had some success, or am attending a special event, I will eat whatever I want.

Once I compiled this personal evaluation, I then made a second list of what these specifications meant for my plan. For instance: one of the most popular diet plans right now incorporates bread products two and three times a day. Automatically, I know this diet won't work for me, because of my gluten and insulin sensitivity. Also, I know that my gallbladder issues make a high-fat paleo or no-carb diet almost impossible because I need to limit fatty foods. And because I'm apple-shaped, I know that I am battling visceral fat, and from what I've read, it tends to surround some vital organs, which is reason enough to undertake a healthier lifestyle.

Ugh, so many factors stand in my way. Should I just give up? No way, baby! Now, it was time to study my inventory and start designing a plan only for me.

Goal Establishment

You know your body, your needs, your Achilles heels. You are now ready to start thinking about your goals.

Of course, we all admire/envy those celebrity women whose bodies bounce back just a few weeks after delivering. We've all seen them, splashing around in the waves on the beach in a string bikini while their newborn is at home with the nanny. (That's mean but probably right. I'm judgy.) They are out there hoping to be photographed by the paparazzi because the public is obsessed with this phenomenon. Is it genetics or have these women starved themselves and camped out in the gym? It's a mystery to us, regular women.

Add the fact that women are waiting for their 30s and even 40s to have children, and you're looking at a new reality of women who are struggling to lose weight. Our bodies don't get all spring back into shape. Because of our fluctuating hormones and slowing metabolisms -- not to mention the processed wheat problems in this world -- there is a generation of women in our 40s who are finding it impossible to move the scale.

I digress.

To finally figure out how to get fit again, it is vital that we set realistic goals for ourselves.

Bikinis are not my goal. It's not necessary to me, at this point. It's more helpful for me to make smaller purposes, to stay honest. And the truth of the matter is, I didn't have rock-hard abs when I was in my glory days, so it's impractical to make them a goal now.

My goal is to feel comfortable in my clothes and to have energy. So, I decided to set my goal on clothing size, rather than a number on the scale. Your weight just doesn't take the whole picture into account. Your muscles weigh more than fat, and there are weeks where you might be retaining water, so in my opinion, it's just not an accurate account of your progress whatsoever. Also, all the constant weighing yourself and seeing no change does NOTHING for your motivation.

Here is how I established my goals:

1. **MEASURE YOURSELF.** One of the first things I did in setting a goal was to get out that old measuring tape and record my starting measurements:

Weight: 171 lbs

Bust: 45."

Waist: 40."

Hips: 44."

Thigh: 24.5."

Arm: 11"

For me, I paid particular attention to the Bust, Waist, Hips numbers, because those were my trouble areas. For you, it might be Hips, Thighs, Arms. As I said, we are all different creatures! There may be a temptation to measure/weigh yourself once a week, but I don't find it helpful at all. Monthly or bi-monthly measuring is best.

2. **GET REAL.** It's time to ask yourself some hard questions. Like, "In the last 5 or 10 years, what weight made me feel the best?" It's not realistic to try to get back to those glory days in our 20s when we could eat anything we wanted and never gain a pound. Our best weight ever is almost irrelevant, if it happened 20 or 25 years ago. It's fantastic if we finally DO wind up there, but in goal setting, it's better to be prudent.

3. **BE SPECIFIC.** It is not enough to say, "I'm going to exercise more." For me, I need to be exact. I need to say, "I'm going to walk for 15 minutes a day after dropping the kids off at school," and go from there. Otherwise, it's too vague of an idea that seems too daunting to accomplish.

4. **REEVALUATE.** It is helpful, after a certain amount of time, to reevaluate your goals. If you're doing well, you could up the ante. If you're struggling, then really look at your program and see where you can improve. Losing weight and staying fit is not a test you take and pass or fail. It's an ongoing process that goes through peaks and valleys. It is not a self-propelling force, however, and does need your attention from time to time.

Visualization and Meditation

Throughout my weight-loss struggles, I have probably thought the following phrase at least a thousand times: "I know what I need to do. So why don't I do it"? Does that sound familiar to you?

The problem is I never went deep enough into my subconscious to make a permanent change. It wasn't something I knew was necessary.

I am willing to bet that half of the people who see this heading skip right past this section. In doing so, they are missing a vital piece of the whole weight puzzle – the mind-body connection. To ignore this component would be setting yourself up for failure.

There are a few cogs of the good weight wheel that are assumed---there need to be dietary changes and a fitness/workout element. But there is another, less-discussed piece of the puzzle that I believe is essential to your success. Without Meditation and Visualization, how will you prepare your mind for the journey you are about to take? It might sound new age-y and right up there with healing crystals and holistic medicine, but when you make an effort, you can train your mind to achieve results. This goes for any of your goals but is especially true for a healthy weight.

Your mind is what decides to eat right or wrong. Your brain chooses to drink more water, to walk on the treadmill, to take the stairs instead of the elevator. And maybe right now, you aren't making those healthy choices for yourself. You can steer yourself toward more robust alternatives.

If you ignore the importance of your mind's involvement, then you are only treating the body. You cannot disconnect frame from memory. I think people know this, to some extent. That is why they hang skinny pictures of themselves on the fridge and pin tons of motivational fitness quotes on Pinterest. They know they must get their brain on board for a healthy weight.

Back in my late teens, I was stricken with panic disorder. Through the help of a counselor, I was introduced to meditation and breathing exercises to help soothe my anxiety. At first, I thought it was all bunk, but after I got over myself and put in the effort, I found that it indeed worked! Because I was so reluctant to try medication, I found that meditation and controlled breathing were just as active, without any side effects.

How does it work? I have no freaking idea. But I decided to take those lessons and apply them to a healthy weight. I sat down at the laptop and wrote a list of reasons why I wanted to lose weight and statements about how I would feel if I were at my ideal weight and body shape. I even went so far as to make a recording of these comments, so that I could meditate on it every morning and prepare myself for a day of good choices.

This is a sample of one of my meditation scripts. Feel free to use this text and edit it to make it your own:

Building Approved Food Lists

You will not read the words "daily menu" anywhere in this book. (Except right there.) Why? Because over the years, I have tried to follow dozens of diet bible daily menus only to wind up feeling defeated and frustrated. Either I didn't like some of the choices offered, or life got in the way, and I didn't have the time to prepare the meals. Maybe I didn't have the expensive, hard-to-find ingredients around the house or the kids wouldn't want to eat what was on the menu. I would start making substitutions, and sooner or later, I wasn't anywhere close to following it anymore. This 'failure' killed my enthusiasm. Before long, I would be eating worse than before.

What finally worked for me was to develop my own, personalized APPROVED FOOD LISTS and a list of RULES. I would make a list of meals that I liked that passed my criteria, followed by list rules that I would support. I made a promise to myself not to put anything in my mouth if it wasn't on the approved list or if it broke a rule. AT LEAST DURING THE LOSING PHASE. This is, without question, the hardest part of my plan. Once I got down to my healthy weight, I would be more lenient. I wasn't going to give up a birthday cake for life. But I was going to stick to the list and the rules until I was satisfied with my physique.

The first step was to go back to my original personal evaluation:

With this information, I am then able to assess specific guidelines for my healthy weight program. For instance, my age alone is of high importance when it comes to deciding what to eat and how to exercise appropriately because it tells me that my estrogen levels are lower than they used to be. Therefore I must watch my carbs. Knowing things like this about myself will help me built my food lists.

But a significant aspect of selecting the proper food to help you get back to a healthy weight is LABEL READING. Without reading labels, how will you know what is right food for you?

When I am grocery shopping, I try to purchase the bulk of my food from the store's outer perimeter: vegetables and fruits, meat and seafood, a bit of dairy. From the other aisles, I keep a close watch on ingredients. If I don't recognize the components, I don't buy it. To keep my liver functioning correctly, it is important to me to keep chemicals out of my diet. The fewer toxins I take in, the less work my liver needs to do. That keeps my liver free to fight disease better. Makes perfect sense to me.

And if we all, collectively, stop buying the garbage that these companies are passing off as 'food,' then perhaps they'll get the message and stop making it. A girl can dream.

I have developed a little cheat sheet that I bring grocery shopping. I know how difficult it can be to remember what you aren't supposed to be eating. Especially in the beginning. Soon, I was able to rattle off every ingredient I should be avoiding. I printed out the cheat sheet, laminated it, and put it in my wallet. One less thing to think about.

Then, I built myself an approved food list. I bought this to the grocery store as well, so that I would purchase the proper foods for myself, and I hung it on my fridge so it was there to remind me what I should be eating. A vital part of this process is to keep the right foods in the home or bring the right foods to work. When bad foods are around, you will be tempted. For myself, it was 'out of sight, out of mind' when it came to the foods I needed to avoid. Luckily, my kids and my husband are good eaters, so they were amenable to healthier foods around the house. Of course, I still kept some of their food around, but as time went on it became more accessible and more accessible to resist.

After creating the approved food lists for myself, I wanted more structure. I wanted a list of accepted MEAL ideas, too, that I could refer to on the fly. As we all know, especially if you're a mom, the day goes by quickly. If you're a stay-home-mom like I am, you know that you barely get done cleaning up after breakfast, and your kid is asking for snack or lunch already. Mealtime takes up a considerable portion of your day. You do NOT want to have to be thinking about acceptable meal ideas when you're time-crunched because you will feel stressed and more likely to revert to meals you know.

After I completed my program, these NEW meals were now part of my routine. I barely even need to refer to my lists anymore. But in the beginning, I was glad to have them. When you're trying to start a new life, you need as much of the work done for you as possible. I needed to remove the 'thinking' out of my program so that my choices would be more automatic. It was the only way to make new habits, and it worked.

What I did was dedicate a folder to my program, which I kept in a drawer in the kitchen. The envelope contained the approved meal list, the approved food list, the nutrition label cheatsheet, and my daily journal. Each day, I would record precisely what I ate, and in the morning, I would refer to the meal list and decide what I would make that day. On grocery shopping day, I would make my file by using the approved food list, and also the journals. It might seem like a lot of work, but it only took a few minutes a day. So worth it!

These are the meal lists I used for myself, one for each phase. But this is something that is very personal. If you were to follow such a program, it would behoove you to create your list of favorite meals that adhere to the requirements. Everyone has their personal tastes!

I want to say that the meal lists contain a lot of recipe-necessary meals, which I don't tend to rely upon for everyday eating. I use my approved meal lists for those times where I need something yummier than my norm – which is mostly a lean protein with some raw veggies of some kind. I might make one of these meals every couple of days. My daily menus are pretty annoying, overall. I don't spend a lot of time on complicated recipes because my time is limited. But once in a while, you need something fun and fancy to spice up your day. Most of my approved meals are relatively straightforward with uncomplicated ingredients, anyway.

NOTE: I highly recommend revisiting your lists at the halfway point, during your recommitment phase. I know that when I reached that point, I had wandered off my lists somewhat, and needed a little adjustment here and there. It's a good time to take off what you didn't like or found too much work, and add a new recipe you might have come across.

Portion Control

Deciding how much food our body needs to survive and thrive is probably one of the most important changes you will need to make, second only to WHAT you're eating.

As you know, Americans are guilty of overeating. Somewhere along the line, we started increasing our portion sizes to the point where a single meal could efficiently deliver more calories/fat/carbs/sodium than you should consume in a single day. Restaurants attract people with giant plates of food, which would have been acceptable if we dined out once a month. But many people are eating out more than twice a week. Some people are dining out once a day! Our bodies are just not meant to process that much food. Especially since we have become the most sedentary people on the planet.

Personally, I knew that controlling my portions was going to be a struggle. Food was a comfort to me, and I liked nothing more than a heaping bowl of spaghetti with buttered bread, or a giant 3-egg omelet packed with pork roll and cheese with a side of home fries and toast. Of course, I washed it all down with a diet soda. I would walk away from the table feeling stuffed and tired, bloated and nauseated. But that never stopped me from eating this way over and over and over and over.

I wasn't listening to my body anymore. If you have children or are around children, you will notice that typically, they eat only when they are hungry and stop eating when they're full. Then they run around for a half-hour. I call my kids 'grazers' because instead of eating three big meals a day, they would eat a little, snack a bit here and there. And they never quit moving. Kids instinctively listen to their bodies signals. Somewhere along the line, I stopped hearing mine.

I know for me, my emotional craving for food was louder than my actual physiological need for food. The signal that should have told me to stop eating was suppressed by the more dominant need to soothe my stress. Food for me was the highlight of my day, especially when my day became consumed with crying babies and sleepless nights. I knew I was overeating. Our bodies are letting us know with bloating and gas and nausea that we've overeaten. But I just wasn't listening, for some reason. I was in denial.

My ambition was to conquer this obstacle, which I knew was not going to be easy. It was a habit that would prove the hardest to break, but once your body becomes used to smaller portions, it is AMAZING how much better you feel, and how easy it is to eat less. Because I was having trouble 'hearing' those signals from my body, I had to retrain myself to recognize the signal for when I'm hungry, and the signal for when I'm full. Sounds easy enough, right?

Some of you might hear the phrase 'eat less' and start to panic. But my objective was not to starve myself or eat less than I needed. I aimed to discover precisely what food my body required, no more, no less. I refused to feel hungry or deprived. I knew there was a middle ground, and I was determined to find mine.

Let's start with the signal that lets us know we're hungry. If you're a meal-skipper, you probably know what hungry feels like, because around 10:30 a.m., you might feel your stomach growling. You never want to wait until you're dizzy, shaky and cranky. This is your body saying, "Hello? I made your stomach growl an hour ago, and you didn't feed me!!" That's why you get ravenous. That is your body's way of saving itself. You didn't listen to your stomach growl, so it went the next step, and now you're eating whatever you can get your hands on, which is probably a donut from the break room or pizza from last night's dinner.

I know for myself that skipping meals is never a good idea because I tend to overeat when I finally get around to feeding myself. Breakfast is a must, for me. So, here is where some people might run into trouble getting in touch with their bodies' signals: maybe you need to eat breakfast to ward off the overeating frenzy later in the day, but you're not hungry in the morning. Don't think I am ignorant of the contradiction I'm making, here. For me, I need to eat breakfast, even if I'm not feeling hunger pains, to avoid a woozy spell later on. It's not often that I don't feel hungry in the morning, however.

The hunger signal starts off subtle. If you eat before you get too hungry, you will be in much better control of what you eat.

The full signal is much harder to get in touch with.

There are lots of variables in play, here. First and foremost, we are usually eating something we like. Unlike when you're a kid, and you have to eat your mom's ghoulish, we typically prepare foods that we like. So, when you're eating something that tastes good, you don't want to stop. Another factor that might come into play is your apprehension about wasting food. Maybe you were always taught to clean your plate, which might be a lifelong habit. These days, life is a lot different regarding how and when we eat. Often, you might find your family eating in front of the TV instead of at the table, and it's much harder to hear your full signal when you're concentrating on whatever show you're watching.

To retrain me to receive and identify these signals was no easy task. It required me to slow down and be more mindful. In the past, I would just grab whatever looked good and as much of it as I wanted. But now, I try to stop, listen to my body, and eat (or not eat) accordingly. I've had to make meal and snack time less automatic, to break the bad habits I'd collected over the years.

The next hurdle was to understand the difference between 'hunger' and 'appetite.' Hunger is a physical need or mechanism of our bodies to ensure we stay alive, whereas appetite is developed as a sensory or psychological reaction to a stimulus (if you see a yummy picture of food on Pinterest or smell sugar cookies baking in the kitchen). They are very different things, and once you make the distinction, you are one step closer to recognizing your hunger signals. I ask myself now, "Am I hungry, or is this an appetite reaction?" Hunger is satisfied with one, regular-sized portion. Appetite is what often persuades you to take a second serving. Or a third.

To gain portion control, I had to develop portion size rules for myself. For breakfast and lunch, I would use a small plate, and plan on a smaller portion of protein with healthy fat and maybe a tiny part of low G.I. carb, like one slice of whole grain bread. I would try to add some raw vegetable to each meal, like sliced tomatoes with a poached egg, or chicken over lettuce for lunch.

The key is to be able to eyeball the permissible portion sizes and stick to it. You will be amazed at how much better you'll feel, just from this simple change.

Even if you never lose a pound, your body will thank you for not clogging it up (and therefore, bogging it down) with food that it just doesn't need.

At times people believe that unhealthy behaviors will not harm them. Young adults have the attitude that "I can smoke now, and in a few years I'll quit before it causes any damage." Unfortunately, nicotine is one of the most addictive drugs known to us, so quitting smoking is not an easy task.

Health problems may arise before you quit, and the risk for lung cancer lingers for years after you stopped. Another example is drinking and driving. The feeling of "I'm in control" or "I can handle it" while under the influence of alcohol is a deadly combination.

Others perceive low risk when engaging in harmful behaviors with people they like for example, sex with someone you've recently met and feel attracted to but see themselves at risk just by being in the same classroom with an HIV-infected person.

Tip to initiate change: No one is immune to sickness, disease, and tragedy. The younger you are when you implement a healthy lifestyle, the better are your odds to attain a long and healthy life. Thus, initiating change right now will help you enjoy the best possible quality of life for as long as you live.

Conclusion

I see you've made it all the way to the end of my book Over 40 and Still Hot. I'm so glad you enjoyed it enough to get all the way through!

How can I guarantee you will have continued success?

I can't.

But you can.

I can give you the strategies I use and these work for me. I encourage you to use them and slightly adapt if you need.

However, a good recipe is a good recipe!

I think a great way to stay on track is to have a clear goal.

When to reset /reassess continue to do x for results.

Write it down. Write down your success plan.

What's your next occasion you want to look great for, to be well for, to be agile for?

Ensure your goals are measurable and realistic. It's great to have short-term goals like events alone, or with friends and groups to aim towards.

For the long term, it can be gratifying to aim for permanent shifts and habits. This doesn't mean once you've reached your weight loss goals you don't get to treat yourself/get to have cheat day/meal. Once achieved, you will have new things you want to meet. There will always be something to work towards, and you will never fully arrive. There will be a new something to strive for... But I think that's half the fun!

Made in the USA
Middletown, DE
01 May 2018